Infectious Diseases Annual Volume 2022

Edited by Katarzyna Garbacz, Tomas Jarzembowski, Yuping Ran, Amidou Samie and Shailendra K. Saxena

Published in London, United Kingdom

Infectious Diseases Annual Volume 2022
http://dx.doi.org/10.5772/intechopen.109247
Edited by Katarzyna Garbacz, Tomas Jarzembowski, Yuping Ran, Amidou Samie and Shailendra K. Saxena

Contributors
Adnan Al-Lahham, Alwyn Rapose, Gokul Shankar Sabesan, Ranjit Singh Aja, Ranjith Mehenderkar, Basanta Kumar Mohanty, Irina A. Rakityanskaya, Tatiana S. Ryabova, Anastasiya A. Kalashnikova, Aklilu Alemayehu, Jacob Bueno de Mesquita, Sirida Youngchim

First published in London, United Kingdom, 2022 by IntechOpen
IntechOpen is the global imprint of INTECHOPEN LIMITED, registered in England and Wales, registration number: 11086078, 5 Princes Gate Court, London, SW7 2QJ, United Kingdom

British Library Cataloguing-in-Publication Data
A catalogue record for this book is available from the British Library

Additional hard and PDF copies can be obtained from orders@intechopen.com

Infectious Diseases Annual Volume 2022
Edited by Katarzyna Garbacz, Tomas Jarzembowski, Yuping Ran, Amidou Samie and Shailendra K. Saxena
p. cm.

This title is part of the Infectious Diseases Book Series, Volume 15
Series Editor: Alfonso J. Rodriguez-Morales

Print ISBN 978-1-83768-943-9
Online ISBN 978-1-83768-944-6
eBook (PDF) ISBN 978-1-83768-945-3
ISSN 2631-6188

IntechOpen Book Series
Infectious Diseases
Volume 15

Aims and Scope of the Series

This series will provide a comprehensive overview of recent research trends in various Infectious Diseases (as per the most recent Baltimore classification). Topics will include general overviews of infections, immunopathology, diagnosis, treatment, epidemiology, etiology, and current clinical recommendations for managing infectious diseases. Ongoing issues, recent advances, and future diagnostic approaches and therapeutic strategies will also be discussed. This book series will focus on various aspects and properties of infectious diseases whose deep understanding is essential for safeguarding the human race from losing resources and economies due to pathogens.

Meet the Series Editor

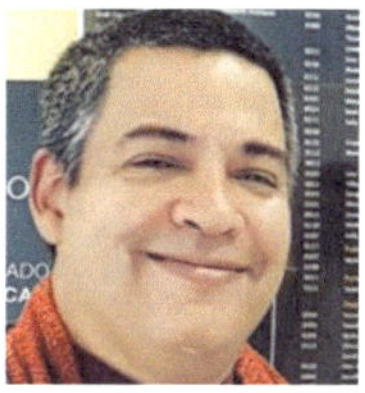

Dr. Rodriguez-Morales is an expert in tropical and emerging diseases, particularly zoonotic and vector-borne diseases (especially arboviral diseases). He is the president of the Travel Medicine Committee of the Pan-American Infectious Diseases Association (API), as well as the president of the Colombian Association of Infectious Diseases (ACIN). He is a member of the Committee on Tropical Medicine, Zoonoses, and Travel Medicine of ACIN. He is a vice-president of the Latin American Society for Travel Medicine (SLAMVI) and a Member of the Council of the International Society for Infectious Diseases (ISID). Since 2014, he has been recognized as a Senior Researcher, at the Ministry of Science of Colombia. He is a professor at the Faculty of Medicine of the Fundacion Universitaria Autonoma de las Americas, in Pereira, Risaralda, Colombia. He is an External Professor, Master in Research on Tropical Medicine and International Health, Universitat de Barcelona, Spain. He is also a professor at the Master in Clinical Epidemiology and Biostatistics, Universidad Científica del Sur, Lima, Peru. In 2021 he has been awarded the "Raul Isturiz Award" Medal of the API. Also, in 2021, he was awarded with the "Jose Felix Patiño" Asclepius Staff Medal of the Colombian Medical College, due to his scientific contributions to COVID-19 during the pandemic. He is currently the Editor in Chief of the journal Travel Medicine and Infectious Diseases. His Scopus H index is 47 (Google Scholar H index, 68).

Meet the Topic Editors

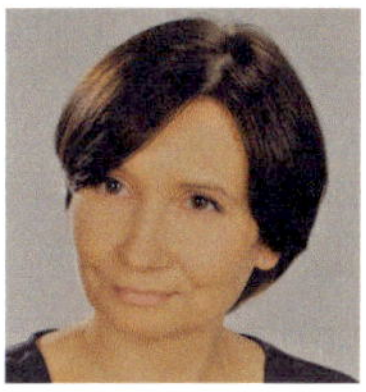

Katarzyna Maria Garbacz, MD, is an Associate Professor at the Medical University of Gdańsk, Poland and she is the head of the Department of Oral Microbiology of the Medical University of Gdańsk. She has published more than 50 scientific publications in peer-reviewed journals. She has been a project leader funded by the National Science Centre of Poland. Prof. Garbacz is a microbiologist working on applied and fundamental questions in microbial epidemiology and pathogenesis. Her research interest is in antibiotic resistance, host-pathogen interaction, and therapeutics development for staphylococcal pathogens, mainly Staphylococcus aureus, which causes hospital-acquired infections. Currently, her research is mostly focused on the study of oral pathogens, particularly Staphylococcus spp.

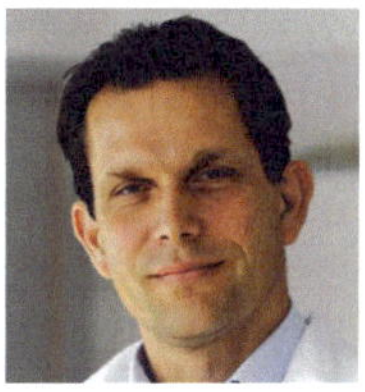

Tomasz Jarzembowski was born in 1968 in Gdansk, Poland. He obtained his Ph.D. degree in 2000 from the Medical University of Gdańsk. After a specialization in clinical microbiology in 2003, he started studying biofilm formation and antibiotic resistance at the single-cell level. In 2015, he obtained his D.Sc. degree. His later study in cooperation with experts in nephrology and immunology resulted in the designation of the new diagnostic method of UTI, patented in 2017. He is currently working at the Department of Microbiology, Medical University of Gdańsk (GUMed), Poland. He is a member of the steering committee of the Gdańsk branch of the Polish Society of Microbiologists and a member of ESCMID. He is also a reviewer and a member of the editorial boards of a number of international journals.

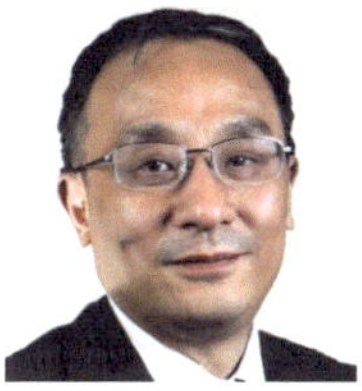

Yuping Ran, Professor, Department of Dermatology, West China Hospital, Sichuan University, Chengdu, China, completed the course in Medical Mycology at the Centraalbureau voor Schimmelcultures, Fungal Biodiversity Centre, Netherlands (2006). He is an International Union of Microbiological Societies fellow, an International Emerging Infectious Diseases fellow, and Centers for Diseases Control and Prevention fellow, in Atlanta, USA. He holds a diploma in Dermatology from the Japanese Society for Investigative Dermatology and a Ph.D. from Juntendo University, Japan. He is the chair of the Sichuan Medical Association Dermatology Committee and was a general secretary of the 19th Annual Meeting of the Chinese Society of Dermatology and the Asia Pacific Society for Medical Mycology (2013). He is in charge of the Annual Medical Mycology Course for over 20 years authorized by the National Continued Medical Education Committee of China. He is also a member of the board of directors of the Asia-Pacific Society for Medical Mycology, associate editor of Mycopathologia, vice-chief of the editorial board of the Chinese Journal of Mycology, and a Board Member and Chair of Mycology Group of Chinese Society of Dermatology.

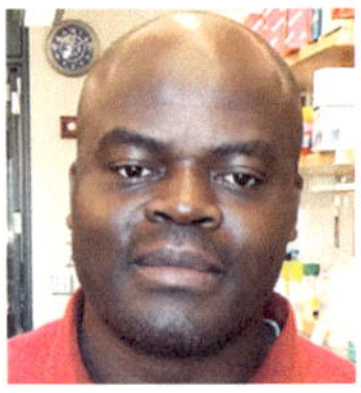

Amidou Samie is an Associate Professor of Microbiology at the University of Venda, in South Africa, where he graduated with his Ph.D. in May 2008. He joined the Department of Microbiology the same year and has been giving lectures on topics covering parasitology, immunology, molecular biology and industrial microbiology. He is currently a rated researcher by the National Research Foundation of South Africa in category C2. He has published widely in the field of infectious diseases and has overseen several MScs and PhDs. His research activities mostly cover topics on infectious diseases from epidemiology to control. His particular interest lies in the study of intestinal protozoan parasites and opportunistic infections among HIV patients as well as the potential impact of childhood diarrhoea on growth and child development. He also conducts research on water-borne diseases and water quality and is involved in the evaluation of point-of-use water treatment technologies using silver and copper nanoparticles in collaboration with the University of Virginia, USA. He also studies the use of medicinal plants for the control of infectious diseases as well as antimicrobial drug resistance.

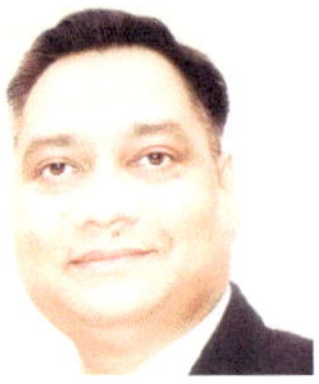

Shailendra K. Saxena is a vice dean and professor at King George's Medical University, Lucknow, India. His research interests involve understanding the molecular mechanisms of host defense during human viral infections and developing new predictive, preventive, and therapeutic strategies for them using Japanese encephalitis virus (JEV), HIV, and emerging viruses as a model via stem cell and cell culture technologies. His research work has been published in various high-impact factor journals (Science, PNAS, Nature Medicine) with a high number of citations. He has received a number of awards and honors in India and abroad including various Young Scientist Awards, BBSRC India Partnering Award, and Dr. JC Bose National Award of the Department of Biotechnology, Min. of Science and Technology, Govt. of India. Prof. Saxena is a fellow of various international societies/academies including the Royal College of Pathologists, United Kingdom; Royal Society of Medicine, London; Royal Society of Biology, United Kingdom; Royal Society of Chemistry, London; and Academy of Translational Medicine Professionals, Austria. He was named a Global Leader in Science by The Scientist. He is also an international opinion leader/expert in vaccination for Japanese encephalitis by IPIC (UK).

Contents

Preface

Streptococci are facultatively anaerobic Gram-positive bacteria that are isolated in large numbers from most human body sites. They are common colonizers of the mucosae. The border between pathogenic and non-pathogenic streptococcal species is often indistinct. Many pathogenic streptococci, such as *Streptococcus pneumoniae*, *Streptococcus pyogenes* may asymptomatically colonize the nasopharynx of healthy people and become a source of endogenous infection under favorable conditions. Streptococcal infection is a complex multi-stage process involving, on the one hand, a host with an array of protective mechanisms of defense, and bacteria with virulence factors that neutralize the above mentioned mechanisms (envelopes, enzymes, toxins, and superantigens) on the other. The predominance of one side or another is reflected by the elimination of the bacteria or infection, either symptomatic or limited to asymptomatic carriage. The clinical course and severity of infection vary greatly among infecting streptococcal strains. Effective ways to prevent both asymptomatic streptococcal colonization and infection, which include vaccination, are constantly demanded.

The Bacterial Infectious Diseases topic features two chapters this year and we look forward to more in the next.

Katarzyna Garbacz and Tomas Jarzembowski
Medical University of Gdańsk,
Gdańsk, Poland
Topic Editors: Bacterial Infectious Diseases

The Fungal Infectious Diseases topic highlights two chapters, the first titled Talaromyces marneffei *Infection: Virulence Factors and Rapid Diagnostics* and the second one titled *Evolution of Parasitism and Pathogenic Adaptations in Certain Medically Important Fungi*. In this first year of its existence, after the topic structure has been introduced, perhaps this is not much but it will, all in all, contribute to this topic's relevance and hopefully open new possible research paths for further novel developments in this particular area which will be welcomed.

Yuping Ran
Sichuan University,
Chengdu, China
Topic Editor: Fungal Infectious Diseases

Parasitic diseases have evolved alongside their human hosts. In many cases, these diseases have adapted so well that they have developed efficient resilience methods in the human host and can live in the host for years. In the current atmosphere of the Coronavirus pandemic, communities around the world, particularly those in different underdeveloped areas, are faced with the growing challenges of the high burden of parasitic diseases which should not be neglected in this context.

Therefore, we need to revisit certain topics in this particular field of research with fresh findings and new perspectives. All researchers are invited to actively participate in this open call.

Amidou Samie
University of Venda,
Thohoyandou, South Africa
Topic Editor: Parasitic Infectious Diseases

The discovery of viruses dates back to around 3700 BC, when the first written record of virus infection was immortalized through representation in Egyptian hieroglyphs, depicting the classical signs of poliomyelitis and smallpox infection. However, the struggle of the human brain with these microbes is still fresh and unanswered. The scientific studies of viruses began in the late 19th century when their existence was documented and the term "virus" was coined. By mid-20th century, almost 2,000 recognized species of animal, plant, and bacterial viruses had been discovered. Despite several achievements over the past years in virology, viruses still continue to pose bigger, new, and fatal threats to the world's populations which poses several challenges to virologists all over the world. Several viral infections that may be fatal or debilitating threaten the human race. The majority of viral diseases attack infants and young children, while others strike people in their prime. There is a continual trend of extreme variation in viral epidemics considering their extent, severity, duration, appearance, reappearance, and the emergence of new diseases.

However, as we develop newer techniques, the viruses are getting smarter, and their advances and abilities to adapt and resist are posing greater challenges to virologists all over the world. The pattern and profile of viral infections are undergoing several changes that make them hard to analyze. Recent outbreaks and resurgence of highly pathogenic viruses continue to dominate the disease incidence rates globally. The need of the hour is to win over the virus, which is not a one step phenomenon; instead, it is a chained and linked process between individuals, researchers, analysts, antiviral drug developers, the government, and the public. However, the effort of opening several hundreds of new labs is appreciated, but viral research needs an upgrade which may be fulfilled by building capacity at various levels. There is an urgent need for learned and trained human resources in virology. Therefore, specialized virology programs should be included at various institutes/universities, as well as medical courses for clinical/medical/basic microbiologists and paramedical staff, to train them in differential and molecular diagnostics/antiviral drug research, etc. In spite of accurate diagnostics, the lack of specific antiviral drugs and vaccines is a major concern, through which emerging, reemerging, and drug-resistant viruses pose the foremost threat. Therefore, there is a desperate need for the development of effective antivirals and vaccine strategies. We should consider another challenging and emerging clinical area of personalized medicines, due to differences in host genetic factors and viral strain variation when compared to foreign countries. A viral outbreak forecast system which can predict viral epidemics/pandemics based on intensive research and molecular biomarkers could be developed, potentially saving thousands of lives nationwide.

The aim of this topic is to collect a comprehensive overview of recent research trends and discoveries in various viral infectious diseases emerging around the globe. The emergence of any viral disease is hard to anticipate, which often contributes to death rates. A viral disease can be defined as an infectious disease that has recently emerged in a population or that exists in nature with a rapid increase in incidence or a geographic range. This topic's aim is to publish work focused on various crucial factors related to emerging viral infectious diseases, including epidemiology, pathogenesis, host immune response, clinical manifestations, diagnosis, treatment, and clinical recommendations for managing viral infectious diseases, highlighting the recent issues with future directions for effective therapeutic strategies.

I am overwhelmed in all humbleness and gratefulness to acknowledge my depth to all the contributors who trusted me and supported me in this work. My research fellows are the motivating force behind anything constructive that I do and a center of my research and academic work. I would like to express my special thanks of gratitude to my mentors, teachers, and students. Also, I would like to thank my colleagues, family, and friends who gave a lot of encouragement and support during the work on this topic. A happy environment at home is essential for any kind of growth, and I thank my family, especially my wife and children for the same.

Shailendra K. Saxena
King George's Medical University,
Lucknow, India
Topic Editor: Viral Infectious Diseases

Section 1

Bacterial Infectious Diseases

Chapter 1

Pneumococcal Carriage in Jordanian Children and the Importance of Vaccination

Adnan Al-Lahham

Abstract

Pneumococcal carriage is a prerequisite for invasive and non-invasive infections, where children and elderly are the most vulnerable groups. Aims: Determine rates of carriage, resistance, and coverage of the pneumococcal conjugate vaccines (PCVs) in children attending day care centers (DCC) in north Jordan. Methods: Nasopharyngeal swabs (NP) were taken from healthy Jordanian children from north Jordan with ages ranging from 1 month to 14 years in the period from 2008 to 2019. Classical methods were used for cultivation, identification, resistance testing, and serotyping. Results: 1866 NP swabs were tested with carriage rate 39.3% (733 isolates). Resistance was variable; however, it showed highest rates for penicillin (89.3%) and trimethoprim-sulfamethoxazole (73.0%). Serotype 19F predominates with 17.6% of all serotypes. Coverage of the future PCV20 was 73.1% compared to the old PCV7 (41.7%). About 493 cases had a previous 1–3 PCV7 injections, among which 256 (51.9%) cases were pneumococcal carriers, distributed as non-PCV vaccine serotypes (31.6%), and with PCV types (68.4%). Conclusions: The potential inclusion of the PCV vaccination in the national immunization program of the country is necessary.

Keywords: *Streptococcus pneumoniae*, PCVs, coverage, nasopharyngeal carriage, resistance

1. Introduction

1.1 Describing the Jordanian situation

Jordan is an upper middle-income country with a total population of 10,806,000 inhabitants, where 44.3% of them are under the age of 19 years, and quite youthful with almost 75% under the age of 30. However, risk groups are the children below 15 years of age (34.4%), among which 11.1% are under the age of 5 years, and 3.67% are over 65 years of age. These age groups (children and elderly) are considered to be at risk from pneumococcal infections globally [1–3]. The prevalence of pneumococcal carriage was the only way in Jordan to detect the serotypes rotating in the Jordanian community, which reflects the clones of infections that might take place. The carriage rates in these areas were relatively high compared to other countries in the region. However, different serotypes were found in different areas. All of these isolates have high resistance rates and are covered to a high percentage with the PCV13 or PCV20. This implies the necessity for a "strategic plan for vaccination in Jordan". *Streptococcus pneumoniae* is considered a leading causative agent of death because of pneumonia globally, especially in the developing countries or in Africa and Asia. In the case and history of Jordan, there is no data available on the pneumococcal infections or serotypes of invasive pneumococcal diseases (IPD), although parts of some publications have described infections with the pneumococci. However, to-date, the PCVs are not available in the National Immunization Program (NIP) of the country, but they are available in the private sector since the year 2000, followed by PCV13 in the year 2010. In Jordan, an average of 400–500 meningitis infections of different causative agents were reported annually, and many infections of otitis media and pneumonia with no identified causative agents, therefore surveillance of the carriage due to *Streptococcus pneumoniae* is essential. Another serious problem for Jordan is the antibiotic consumption, where no reported data are available. Although Jordan is one of the best countries in the region for medical tourism, but there is no numbers stating the antibiotic consumption of the country, where high resistance rates in antibiotics were found [4]. Causes for the high antibiotic resistance in the country are the misuse and abuse of the antibiotics [5, 6]. Furthermore, there are no statistics from the Ministry of Health (MOH) of Jordan regarding the statistics of IPD taking place in hospitals. However, only non-meningococcal meningitis is registered from the statistical department of the MOH, which includes a variety of causative agents including *Streptococcus pneumoniae* (i.e., pneumococcus). This fact is shown in **Figure 1** from the year 1990–2018. By checking these data in the figure, it appears that more than 50% of all cases are from Irbid (North Jordan), 1% from Madaba and 10% from Amman. However, almost 20% of the causative agents of non-meningococcal meningitis are due to the pneumococcus [7]. Another crucial point about Jordan is the absence of national centers working separately on different types of bacteria. These centers in the developed countries and other countries work together with the epidemiological national centers to develop statistics about the rate of invasive diseases caused by infectious agents and their resistance development. Such data are important for setting recommendations to develop new anti-infectious products or to set new treatment strategies. Furthermore, collection

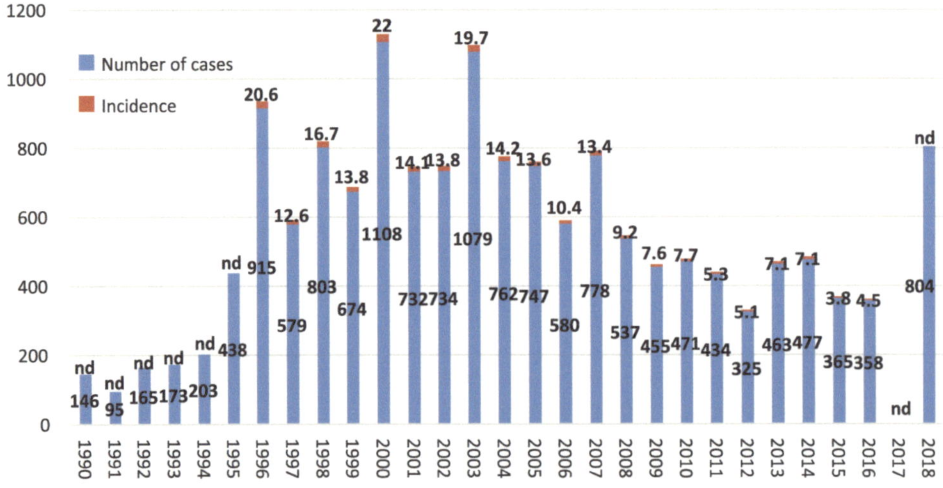

Figure 1.
Number of cases and incidence/100,000 of non-meningococcal meningitis in Jordan.

of invasive samples isolated at the hospitals is almost impossible, because the patients have consumed antibiotics prior to the microbiological sample testing. Therefore, shifting the surveillance to study the carriage of the pneumococci in children was the solution to find out all the possible serotypes rotating with their resistance data.

1.2 Global importance of *Streptococcus pneumoniae* (i.e., the pneumococcus)

S. pneumoniae, or the pneumococcus, is a lancet shape, Gram-positive diplococci, bile soluble, mainly optochin sensitive, and encapsulated. The diversity of capsular types is large, with more than 100 serotypes recognized to date based on the composition of the capsular polysaccharide. Many *S. pneumoniae* serotypes are capable of causing invasive diseases, including meningitis, septicemia, bacteremia, and non-invasive diseases like pneumonia, sinusitis and others; however, most of these diseases globally are caused by a small number of common serotypes [8]. The relative contribution of each serotype to the local burden of disease varies globally, with serotypes 1, 5, 23F, 19A, 19F, 6B and 6A more prominent in developing countries. *S. pneumoniae* infections may vary seasonally and large outbreaks exists but rarely found [8–10]. Meningitis due to *S. pneumoniae* occurs most commonly in early ages of children and in patients over 65 years of age, with an estimated incidence rate of 17 cases per 100,000 population in children less than five years of age [11]. This bacterium is widely spread and can also be found in pets [12]. As a comparison, the incidence of non-meningococcal meningitis for Jordan is estimated to be 4.5/100,000 cases in the year 2016 as shown in the figure. The case fatality rate for meningitis due to *S. pneumoniae* in children less than five years of age exceeds 73% in some parts of the world.

An important study done by the GBD 2016 Lower Respiratory Infections Collaborators in 2016 showed that the lower respiratory infections are the leading cause of morbidity and mortality around the world [13]. This study provides an up-to-date analysis of the burden of lower respiratory infections in 195 countries for the past 26 years, and shows how the burden of lower respiratory infection has changed in people of all ages. Their Findings In 2016 indicate that lower respiratory infections caused 652,572 deaths in children younger than 5 years, 1,080,958 deaths in adults older than 70 years, and 2,377,697 deaths globally in people of all ages. In this regard, *Streptococcus pneumoniae* was the leading cause of lower respiratory infection morbidity and mortality globally, contributing to more deaths than all other etiologies combined in 2016 [13].

S. pneumoniae was given the name as the forgotten killer in children in 2006 by the WHO in 2006 [14]. Furthermore, according to the WHO, 142 countries have introduced the PCV in the National Immunization Program. Jordan as one of the upper middle-income countries has not included this vaccine to the National Immunization Program (NIP) to-date.

The aim of this chapter is to show results of investigations of continuous surveillance on the carriage of *Streptococcus pneumoniae* from 2008 to 2019 in Jordanian children and to show the need of the inclusion of the PCVs in the NIP of the country.

2. Material and methods

Research studies on the carriage of Streptococcus pneumoniae were approved by the Independent Ethical Committee (IEC) of the Ministry of Health (MOH) of Jordan, followed by approval of the Ministry of Health (MOH) with approval number

8/75/2/2257, and other approvals of the directorates of each day care center (DCC). Informed written consent for the participants and the use of NP swabs was obtained from parents prior to collecting the swabs. Parents were educated on the benefits of future vaccination with the available PCVs. Nasopharyngeal swabs were taken from children attending the governmental Day Care Centers (DCCs) from the governorates of Ajlun (n = 415) [15], Madaba (n = 761) [1, 16], private clinic in Amman (n = 149) [16], Irbid (n = 423) [1], Wadi Alseer (n = 118) [17], with total number of samples 1866. Only one NP-swab was obtained from each child with exception to the research project from Ajlun, where 3 consequent samples were taken at 2 months at the time of the first vaccination, then at 4 months of age at the time of the second vaccination and finally a third sample was taken 2–3 months after the third vaccination with PCV7. NP-samples were collected in the period from 2008–2019. Processing, culturing and identification were done by classical methods [1, 18]. Resistance testing was performed according to the latest CLSI standards using *S. pneumoniae* ATCC 49,619 as a control strain [19]. The Neufeld's Quellung reaction method was used for Serotyping using type and factor sera provided by the Statens Serum Institute (SSI), Copenhagen, Denmark.

3. Results and discussion

Four governorates and the capital of Jordan were tested during the whole period of carriage surveillance in Jordan. The total carriage rate for the whole period and for the whole population tested was 39.3% as presented in **Table 1**. The highest carriage rate was in the governorate of Ajlun with 58.1%, because three samples were obtained from the same child over one year period. Nevertheless, this carriage rate of Ajlun was not significantly different ($p > 0.05$) from the carriage rate obtained from Wadi Al Seer, even with only one NP-swab obtained from each child. Wadi Al Seer and Ajlun were tested almost at the same period. The most interesting finding of all cities is the findings in the capital of Amman, where only 13.4% of the children involved in the study were carriers and that the coverage of the PCVs was minimal as found in **Table 1**. This was due to the reason that 69 cases from 149 (46.3%) were vaccinated with PCV7. Only 11 cases from the vaccinated children of Amman were carriers, but none of them was carrier of PCV7 serotype. The second highest carriage was shown in Madaba with 37.1% carriage rate, followed by Irbid with carriage rate of 29.6%. Coverage rates of the PCVs were highest (76.0%) for Irbid with PCV20, and this coverage was not significantly different from the PCV20 coverage for Irbid city ($p < 0.05$). To-date, there are at least 220 publications all over the world investigating carriage or nasopharyngeal carriers of Streptococcus pneumoniae. Our findings are comparable with other studies all over the world; in the region as an example, a study done in Palestine in 2013 has found carriage rates in 11 cities of Palestine to be from 34.1% in Ramallah up to 66.7% in Tubas [20]. In the kingdom of Saudi Arabia, carriage rate was found in 2014 to be 6% [21]. Another study done in 11 countries of Asia and the Middle East on 4963 children below 5 years of age found nasal carriage rate of 22.3% of antibiotic-resistant pneumococci isolates [22]. In Israel, carriage rates tested on ages between 2 and 24 months was shown to increase with age from 2 months with 26% carriage rate to 62% at age of 24 months [23]. In a recent study about carriage of the pneumococcus in Indonesia showed high carriage rate of 73% in school children with acute otitis media (AOM) [24]. Dominant serotypes of the school children were 23A (11 %), 6A/6B (10 %), 3 (8 %), 14 (7 %), 6C/6D (7 %), 11A/11D (6 %), 15B/15C

City	Year from–to	No. of samples	Carriage rate (%)	Coverage of PCV7 (%)	Coverage of PCV10 (%)	Coverage of PCV13 (%)	Coverage of PCV20 (%)
Wadi Al Seer	Mar. 2008–Nov. 2009	118	55.1	52.3	52.3	58.5	73.0
Ajlun	Jun. 2009–Nov. 2010	415	58.1	32.1	32.1	50.4	70.9
Amman	May 2015–Apr. 2016	149	13.4	5	5	10	35
Irbid	Dec. 2017–Mar. 2019	423	29.6	51.2	51.2	65.6	76.0
Madaba	May 2015–Mar. 2019	761	37.3	50.7	51.1	65.1	75.7
Total	Mar. 2008–Mar. 2019	1866	39.3	42.4	42.7	58.4	72.4

Table 1.
Carriage rate of S. pneumoniae *in 5 cities of Jordan with the coverage rate of PCVs including the future PCV20.*

(4 %) and 35 B (4 %). Coverage of the PCV13 in the Indonesian study was 41%. Other study in south Italy on healthy children aged 1–7 years attending day-care centers and schools showed nasopharyngeal colonization rate of Streptococcus pneumoniae to be 18.29%. PCV13 serotypes of this study covered 60.34% of the isolates with serotypes 19A, 19F, 14, 6B, or 23F; and that 8.62% of the strains were intermediately resistant to penicillin, 65.5% were erythromycin-resistant, and 17.2% were resistant to Co-trimoxazole [25]. To date, there is no data describing the invasive Streptococcus pneumoniae infections in Jordan, but this bacterium was identified as the causative agent in 30% of meningitis cases in Yemen, 16% in the UAE, 19–21% in Kuwait, 13% in Qatar, 23–31% in Saudi Arabia, and 21–30% in Egypt [26].

Resistance rates to antibiotics are increasing worldwide. The main reasons for this global threat of resistance are the misuse and abuse of the antibiotics [27]. Streptococcus pneumoniae is one of the major pathogens of community-acquired respiratory tract infections, where Alexander Project in 1997 for resistance showed the variation of antibiotic resistance in Europe [28]. In our studied 5 regions in Jordan as found in **Table 2**, resistance rates to penicillin varied from 80% to 95.4%, and for erythromycin from 55% to 73.6%, for clindamycin from 20%–44.4%, and for Co-trimoxazole (SXT) from 30%–78.5%. Extreme differences in antibiotic resistance were observed in this surveillance in the last 13 years. This resistance is increasing in Europe and in the United states [29, 30]. More than 80% of the resistance is covered by the new PCV20 [27].

In **Table 3**, an uneven distribution of the serotypes in each city was found. Certain clones of the serotypes were found only in one city or two, but not in others. As an example, Serotype 5 was only found in Madaba. This serotype 5 is prevalent in many countries [31–35]. Serotype 4 was only found in Ajlun, but it is also prevalent in many countries as causative agent of an outbreak in a home for aged people [36, 37]. Serotype 13 was also only found in Ajlun, which was found as multidrug resistant in Russia [38]. Serotypes 19A and 19F were mainly found in Ajlun and Madaba.

Table 4 gives an insight about the differences and comparisons of the Jordanian carriage rate, resistance and coverage of PCVs with other countries worldwide. In literature, pneumococcal nasopharyngeal carriage was studied in different directions,

City	No. of isolates	% PEN R	% ERY R	% CLI R	% TET R	% SXT R	% CHA R
Wadi Al Seer	63/118	80.0	61.5	33.8	53.8	73.8	9.5
Ajlun	241/415	82.0	55.7	36.3	46.8	62.3	2.5
Amman	20/149	90.0	55.0	20.0	45.0	30.0	0.0
Irbid	125/423	86.3	75.0	30.8	45.5	68.6	2.4
Madaba	284/761	95.4	73.6	44.4	52.8	78.5	3.7
Total	733/1866	89.4	64.8	36.3	47.6	73.0	3.1

Abbreviations: PEN (Penicillin), ERY (Erythromycin), CLI (Clindamycin), TET (Tetracycline), SXT (Sulfamethoxazole-Trimethoprim), CHA (Chloramphenicol), R (Resistance).

Table 2.
Resistance rate of S. pneumoniae in 5 cities of Jordan.

Serotype	Total no. (%)	Ajlun no.	Wadi Al Seer no.	Amman no.	Irbid no.	Madaba no.
3	12 (1.6%)	4	0	0	1	7
4	1 (0.14%)	1	0	0	0	0
5	1 (0.14%)	0	0	0	0	1
13	1 (0.14%)	1	0	0	0	0
14	40 (5.5%)	9	2	0	9	20
21	1 (0.14%)	1	0	0	0	0
28A	8 (1.1%)	1	0	0	1	6
34	4 (0.55%)	0	2	0	0	2
42	1 (0.14%)	1	0	0	0	0
10A	10 (1.4%)	4	0	0	1	5
10F	1 (0.14%)	1	0	0	0	0
11A	44 (6.0%)	21	3	3	4	13
15A	19 (2.6%)	10	3	1	3	2
15B	23 (3.1%)	13	1	0	3	6
15C	17 (2.3%)	6	0	0	5	6
15F	1 (0.14%)	0	1	0	0	0
16A	2 (0.27%)	0	0	0	0	2
16B	1 (0.14%)	1	0	0	0	0
16F	13 (1.8%)	7	1	0	4	1
17F	12 (1.6%)	4	1	0	1	6
18A	1 (0.14%)	0	1	0	0	0
18C	9 (1.2%)	0	0	0	1	8
19A	38 (5.2%)	19	2	0	4	13
19F	129 (17.6%)	29	12	1	26	61
22A	2 (0.27%)	0	0	0	0	2

Serotype	Total no. (%)	Ajlun no.	Wadi Al Seer no.	Amman no.	Irbid no.	Madaba no.
22F	2 (0.27%)	0	1	1	0	0
23*	5 (0.68%)	0	0	0	1	4
23A	26 (3.5%)	9	2	1	2	12
23B	1 (0.14%)	0	0	0	0	1
23F	59 (8.0%)	11	8	0	15	25
24F	7 (0.95%)	7	0	0	0	0
33A	3 (0.4%)	2	1	0	0	0
33F	7 (0.95%)	6	1	0	0	0
35A	3 (0.4%)	0	1	0	1	1
35B	12 (1.6%)	8	4	0	0	0
35C	1 (0.14%)	1	0	0	0	0
35F	2 (0.27%)	2	0	0	0	0
6A	65 (8.9%)	29	2	1	13	20
6B	58 (7.9%)	14	11	0	12	21
6C	4 (0.55%)	0	0	1	2	1
7B	5 (0.68%)	2	1	0	0	2
7C	1 (0.14%)	1	0	0	0	0
7F	1 (0.14%)	1	0	0	0	0
9N	9 (1.2%)	3	0	3	0	3
9V	9 (1.2%)	3	1	0	1	4
Pool C	6 (0.81%)	0	0	0	5	1
Pool D	2 (0.27%)	0	0	0	1	1
Pool E	4 (0.55%)	0	0	0	2	2
Pool F	1 (0.14%)	0	0	0	1	0
Pool G	9 (1.2%)	0	0	0	1	6
Pool I	6 (0.81%)	0	0	0	1	5
Mixed 14 & 6B	1 (0.14%)	0	0	0	0	1
NT	18 (2.5%)	7	1	0	2	8
Others*	15 (2.0%)	0	0	8	0	7

**Isolates from antisera pools C, D, E, F, G, I, which are not included in the PCVs*

Table 3.
Serotypes detected in the surveillance studies with numbers isolated in each city.

either to find out the carriage rate, to check the impact of the PCVs on colonization, or to check the rate of carriage before and after vaccination strategies, or the carriage rates after certain infection, and many other issues related. The data available in **Table 4** are from the region, from Africa, from Europe, and Latin America. As an example, in Palestine 11 cities were tested for pneumococcal carriage with rates ranging from 34.1% in Ramallah to 77.7% in Salfeet [20].

Country	Study period	Rate of carriage	PEN R (%)	ERY R (%)	CLI R (%)	SXT R (%)	PCV7 coverage	PCV13 coverage	Reference
Jordan	2008/19	39.3	89.4	64.8	36.3	73.0	42.4	58.4	[1, 15–17]
Palestine	2013	55.7	10.9	30.3	nd	45.9	55.7	nd	[20]
Ethiopia	2017	18.4	15.0	23.9	nd	nd	nd	nd	[39]
Turkey	2017	14.0	nd	nd	nd	nd	12.6	nd	[40]
Palestine (EJ)	2014	30.7	nd	nd	nd	nd	47.0	62.0	[41]
Palestine	2014	28.6	nd	nd	nd	nd	41.2	54.8	[41]
Gaza Strip	2009	50.0	70.0	nd	nd	nd	54.0	71.0	[42]
Pakistan	2013	73.6	nd	nd	nd	nd	38.9	53.1	[43]
Gambia	2009	72.0	nd	nd	nd	nd	24.7	46.8	[44]
Finland	1994/95	49.0	nd	nd	nd	nd	nd	nd	[45]
Brazil	2008/09	55	38.4	nd	nd	73.8	nd	nd	[46]

Abbreviations: nd = not defined; PEN (Penicillin), ERY (Erythromycin), CLI (Clindamycin), SXT (Sulfamethoxazole-Trimethoprim), R (Resistance), PCV7 (7-Valent Pneumococcal Conjugate Vaccine), PCV13 (13-valent Pneumococcal Conjugate Vaccine).

Table 4.
Comparison of carriage rate, resistance and coverage of PCV7 and PCV13 in other locations (regional and international).

4. Conclusions

The prevalence of pneumococcal carriage was the only way in Jordan to detect the serotypes rotating in the Jordanian community, which reflects the clones of infections that might take place. The carriage rates in these areas were relatively high compared to other countries in the region. However, different serotypes were found in different areas. All of these isolates have high resistance rates and are covered to a high percentage with the PCV13 or PCV20. This implies the necessity for a strategic plan for vaccination in Jordan.

Acknowledgements

The author would like to thank the supporting institutions for this prevalence including the German Jordanian University, Wyeth (Now Pfizer), and Pfizer. Special thanks for the participating children with their parents, and for the MOH for the approvals to make this study successful.

Conflict of interest

The author declares no conflict of interest.

Author details

Adnan Al-Lahham
Department of Biomedical Engineering, School of Applied Medical Sciences, German Jordanian University, Amman, Jordan

*Address all correspondence to: adnan.lahham@gju.edu.jo

References

[1] Al-Lahham A. Multicenter study of pneumococcal carriage in children 2 to 4 years of age in the winter seasons of 2017-2019 in Irbid and Madaba governorates of Jordan. PLoS One. 2020;**15**(8):e0237247

[2] Fletcher MA, Haridy H. Decline in childhood respiratory-related mortality after the introduction of the pneumococcal conjugate vaccine in Morocco. Journal of Infection and Public Health. 2021;**14**(3):387-388

[3] Fletcher MA et al. Controlling invasive pneumococcal disease: Is vaccination of at-risk groups sufficient? International Journal of Clinical Practice. 2006;**60**(4):450-456

[4] Al-Bakri AG, Bustanji Y, Yousef AM. Community consumption of antibacterial drugs within the Jordanian population: Sources, patterns and appropriateness. International Journal of Antimicrobial Agents. 2005;**26**(5):389-395

[5] Abdel-Qader DH et al. Awareness of antibiotic use and resistance in Jordanian Community. Journal of Primary Care and Community Health. 2020;**11**:1-8

[6] Dar-Odeh NS et al. Antibiotic prescribing practices by dentists: A review. Therapeutics and Clinical Risk Management. 2010;**6**:301-306

[7] Dagan R. Epidemiology of pediatric meningitis caused by Haemophilus influenzae B, Streptococcus pneumoniae and Neisseria meningitidis in Israel. Israel Journal of Medical Sciences. 1994;**30**(5-6):351-355

[8] Johnson HL et al. Systematic evaluation of serotypes causing invasive pneumococcal disease among children under five: The pneumococcal global serotype project. PLoS Medicine. 2010;**7**(10):e1000348

[9] Antonio M et al. Seasonality and outbreak of a predominant Streptococcus pneumoniae serotype 1 clone from The Gambia: Expansion of ST217 hypervirulent clonal complex in West Africa. BMC Microbiology. 2008;**8**:198

[10] Leimkugel J et al. An outbreak of serotype 1 Streptococcus pneumoniae meningitis in northern Ghana with features that are characteristic of Neisseria meningitidis meningitis epidemics. The Journal of Infectious Diseases. 2005;**192**(2):192-199

[11] O'Brien KL et al. Burden of disease caused by Streptococcus pneumoniae in children younger than 5 years: Global estimates. Lancet. 2009;**374**(9693):893-902

[12] van der Linden M et al. Molecular characterization of pneumococcal isolates from pets and laboratory animals. PLoS One. 2009;**4**(12):e8286

[13] Collaborators GLRI. Estimates of the global, regional, and national morbidity, mortality, and aetiologies of lower respiratory infections in 195 countries, 1990-2016: A systematic analysis for the Global Burden of Disease Study 2016. The Lancet Infectious Diseases. 2018;**18**(11):1191-1210

[14] Wardlow TJE, Hodge MJ. World Health Organization, UNICEF, Pneumonia: The forgotten Killer of Children. 2006

[15] Al-Lahham A, Abu Qayyas J, Van der Linden M. The impact of the 7-valent

pneumococcal conjugate vaccine on nasopharyngeal carriage of Streptococcus pneumoniae in infants of Ajlun governorate in Jordan. Jordan. Journal of Biological Sciences. 2018;**11**:155-162

[16] Al-Lahham A et al. Urban and rural disparities in pneumococcal carriage and resistance in Jordanian Children, 2015-2019. Vaccines (Basel). 2021;**9**(7):789

[17] Al-Lahham A, Van der Linden M. Streptococcus pneumoniae carriage, resistance and serotypes among Jordanian children from Wadi Al Seer District, JORDAN. International Arab Journal of Antimicrobial Agents. 2014;**4**(2:5):1-8

[18] Verani JR et al. Nasopharyngeal carriage of Streptococcus pneumoniae among HIV-infected and -uninfected children <5 years of age before introduction of pneumococcal conjugate vaccine in Mozambique. PLoS One. 2018;**13**(2):e0191113

[19] CLSI. Performance Standards for Antimicrobial Susceptibility Testing. 31th ed. USA: Clinical and Laboratory Standards Institute; 2021

[20] Nasereddin A et al. Streptococcus pneumoniae from Palestinian nasopharyngeal carriers: Serotype distribution and antimicrobial resistance. PLoS One. 2013;**8**(12):e82047

[21] Memish ZA et al. Impact of the Hajj on pneumococcal transmission. Clinical Microbiology and Infection. 2015;**21**(1):77

[22] Lee NY et al. Carriage of antibiotic-resistant pneumococci among Asian children: A multinational surveillance by the Asian Network for Surveillance of Resistant Pathogens (ANSORP). Clinical Infectious Diseases. 2001;**32**(10):1463-1469

[23] Dagan R et al. Carriage of resistant pneumococci by children in southern Israel and impact of conjugate vaccines on carriage. Clinical Microbiology and Infection. 1999;**5**(Suppl. 4):S29-S37

[24] Wahyono DJ et al. Nasopharyngeal carriage rates and serotype distribution of Streptococcus pneumoniae among school children with acute otitis media in Central Java, Indonesia. Access Microbiol. 2021;**3**(7):000249

[25] Schettini F Jr et al. Nasopharyngeal colonization of Streptococcus pneumoniae in healthy children: Percentage of carriers, serotypes distribution and antibiotic resistance. Minerva Pediatrica. 2003;**55**(5):439-445

[26] Shibl A, Memish Z, Pelton S. Epidemiology of invasive pneumococcal disease in the Arabian Peninsula and Egypt. International Journal of Antimicrobial Agents. 2009;**33**(5):9

[27] Al-Lahham A. Prevalence of Pneumococcal Carriage among Jordanian Infants in the First 6 Months of Age, 2008-2016. Vaccine. 2021;**9**(11):1283

[28] Adam D. Global antibiotic resistance in Streptococcus pneumoniae. The Journal of Antimicrobial Chemotherapy. 2002;**50**(Suppl):1-5

[29] Appelbaum PC. Resistance among Streptococcus pneumoniae: Implications for drug selection. Clinical Infectious Diseases. 2002;**34**(12):1613-1620

[30] Brueggemann AB, Doern GV. Resistance among Streptococcus pneumoniae: Patterns, mechanisms, interpreting the breakpoints. The American Journal of Managed Care. 2000;**6**(Suppl. 23):S1189-S1196

[31] Dawar M et al. A case of necrotizing fasciitis due to Streptococcus

pneumoniae serotype 5 in Saskatchewan. Canadian Journal of Infectious Diseases and Medical Microbiology. 2008;**19**(1):69-71

[32] Balicer RD et al. Control of *Streptococcus pneumoniae* serotype 5 epidemic of severe pneumonia among young army recruits by mass antibiotic treatment and vaccination. Vaccine. 2010;**28**(34):5591-5596

[33] Romney MG et al. Large community outbreak of Streptococcus pneumoniae serotype 5 invasive infection in an impoverished, urban population. Clinical Infectious Diseases. 2008;**47**(6):768-774

[34] Kobayashi M et al. Pneumococcal serotype 5 colonization prevalence among newly arrived unaccompanied children 1 year after an outbreak-Texas, 2015. The Pediatric Infectious Disease Journal. 2017;**36**(2):236-238

[35] Rolo D et al. Serotype 5 pneumococci causing invasive pneumococcal disease outbreaks in Barcelona, Spain (1997 to 2011). Journal of Clinical Microbiology. 2013;**51**(11):3585-3590

[36] Hava DL, Camilli A. Large-scale identification of serotype 4 *Streptococcus pneumoniae* virulence factors. Molecular Microbiology. 2002;**45**(5):1389-1406

[37] Gleich S et al. *Streptococcus pneumoniae* serotype 4 outbreak in a home for the aged: report and review of recent outbreaks. Infection Control and Hospital Epidemiology. 2000;**21**(11):711-717

[38] Savinova T et al. Multiple-drug resistant nasopharyngeal *Streptococcus pneumoniae* isolated in Russia: Serotypes, antimicrobial susceptibility, and molecular characterization of the emergent serotype 13/ST2754 lineage. Microbial Drug Resistance. 2021;**28**(1):39-47

[39] Abaye G et al. Prevalence and risk factors of pneumococcal nasopharyngeal carriage in healthy children attending kindergarten, in district of Arsi Zone, South East, Ethiopia. BMC Research Notes. 2019;**12**(1):253

[40] Arvas A et al. Pneumococcal nasopharyngeal carriage in young healthy children after pneumococcal conjugate vaccine in Turkey. Balkan Medical Journal. 2017;**34**(4):362-366

[41] Abu Seir R et al. Comparison of early effects of pneumococcal conjugate vaccines: PCV7, PCV10 and PCV13 on *Streptococcus pneumoniae* nasopharyngeal carriage in a population based study; The Palestinian-Israeli Collaborative Research (PICR). PLoS One. 2018;**13**(11):e0206927

[42] Regev-Yochay G et al. Streptococcus pneumoniae carriage in the Gaza strip. PLoS One. 2012;**7**(4):e35061

[43] Nisar MI et al. Nasopharyngeal carriage of *Streptococcus pneumoniae* in children under 5 years of age before introduction of pneumococcal vaccine (PCV10) in urban and rural districts in Pakistan. BMC Infectious Diseases. 2018;**18**(1):672

[44] Usuf E et al. Pneumococcal carriage in rural Gambia prior to the introduction of pneumococcal conjugate vaccine: A population-based survey. Tropical Medicine & International Health. 2015;**20**(7):871-879

[45] Syrjanen RK et al. Nasopharyngeal carriage of *Streptococcus pneumoniae* in Finnish children younger than 2 years old. The Journal of Infectious Diseases. 2001;**184**(4):451-459

[46] Menezes AP et al. Nasopharyngeal carriage of *Streptococcus pneumoniae* among children in an urban setting in Brazil prior to PCV10 introduction. Vaccine. 2016;**34**(6):791-797

Chapter 2

Streptococcal Skin and Skin-Structure Infections

Alwyn Rapose

Abstract

Infections attributable to *Streptococcus* are protean. These range from mild skin and soft tissue infections to life-threatening conditions like meningitis, endocarditis and toxic shock syndrome. In addition, streptococcal infection can be associated with noninfectious sequelae like rheumatic fever and post-streptococcal glomerulonephritis. There is a wide range of *Streptococcus spp.* causing human infections and different classifications of these organisms have been described, the most quoted being the Lancefield classification based on cell-wall antigens. *Streptococci* can be studied based on their species: *S. pyogenes, S. pneumoniae, S. anginosus* etc. or by the Lancefield classification group A, B, C, D etc. or by the clinical syndromes associated with these bacteria. This chapter will describe clinical syndromes associated with streptococcal skin and soft tissue infections ranging from mild: cellulitis and lymphangitis which can be treated in the out-patient setting, to more aggressive manifestations that require hospitalization (sepsis and toxic shock syndrome) and even surgery (necrotizing fasciitis, myositis and gangrene), It will also provide clues to clinical diagnosis as well as suggest recommendations for optimized management of these conditions.

Keywords: *Streptococcus*, Skin and Skin-Structure Infections (SSTI), Necrotizing Fasciitis (NF), Toxic Shock syndrome (TSS)

1. Introduction

Streptococcal skin and skin-structure infection (SSTI) is associated with significant morbidity all over the world and the impact is felt predominantly in resource-poor areas with inadequate personal hygiene and over-crowded living conditions. While exact numbers are difficult to estimate on account of the lack of systematic reporting, a literature search conducted by Sims and colleagues [1] reported an estimated prevalence of 18 million cases, with an incidence rate of around 1.78 million cases per year of invasive *S. pyogenes* (*S. pyogenes*) infection in 2005, and more than 140 million cases of impetigo globally each year as reported in the 2010 Global Burden of Disease study. Rising numbers of cases of infectious diseases of the skin is also seen in Western nations, probably driven by drug abuse and homelessness [2, 3]. Increased cases result in increased costs from emergency room visits and hospital care, hence outpatient parenteral antibiotic therapy (OPAT) has proven to be a valuable alternative to hospitalization [4], and when patients are chosen appropriately, OPAT results in very significant cost-savings without compromising outcomes [5]. Advances in pharmaceutical research has contributed to development of longer acting antibiotics that can be dosed once a day and in some cases once a week. There is ongoing research to determine the optimum duration of antibiotic therapy for these conditions.

Skin infections have been variously classified based on different criteria like depth of infection or the bacterial agents causing the infections or as primary infection in contrast to infection of pre-existing wounds or skin conditions. A very practical classification of patients hospitalized with skin infections (cellulitis versus abscess versus skin infections with additional complicating factors) has been described by Jenkins et al. [6]. The authors found in their study that cutaneous abscesses were primarily caused by *Staphylococcus aureus* and less often by the *Streptococcus spp*, in contrast with cellulitis which was caused primarily by *β-hemolytic streptococci* and less commonly by *Staphylococcus spp*. This differentiation is especially helpful when choosing the appropriate narrow spectrum antibiotic therapy for individual patients with these diagnoses. In contrast, "skin infections with additional complications" require more broad antibiotic coverage on account of mixed bacterial infection or infection with unusual organisms.

The clinical features of common streptococcal SSTIs and the antibiotics used in the management of these conditions will be further elaborated in this chapter.

2. Streptococcal pyoderma

Superficial skin infection has been described as **impetigo or pyoderma**. This is in contrast to more invasive diseases cellulitis and erysipelas. Impetigo (and the less precise term pyoderma) refers to superficial infection that begins in the form of a papule that progresses to a vesicle and pustule, ultimately forming crusted lesions (**Figure 1**). They resolve with hyper or hypopigmentation. These infections are caused either by *Staphylococcus* or *Streptococcus*, and one cannot clinically differentiate between the two causative organisms. They occur as a complication of underlying skin diseases

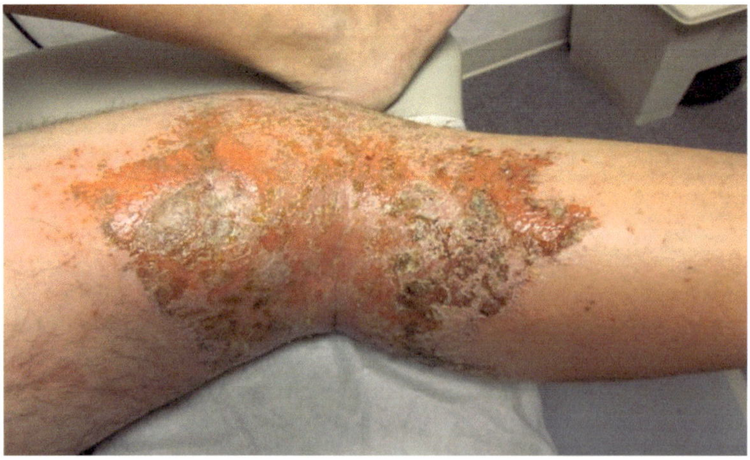

Figure 1.
Impetigo secondary to infected contact dermatitis.

like scabies [1] or contact dermatitis. The streptococci associated with these infections are most often group A (*S. pyogenes*). However other serotypes can also be isolated on cultures from these infections. Although considered benign, these infections could progress to more locally invasive cutaneous diseases (see below) and are associated with post-streptococcal complications like glomerulonephritis and acute rheumatic fever in resource limited populations (as reviewed in other chapters of this textbook).

3. Treatment of impetigo

Antiseptic soaks and antibacterial creams are the mainstay of therapy for impetigo. A wide variety of topical antimicrobial agents are available including silver-based products, iodides, hydrogen peroxide, zinc, chlorhexidine and potassium permanganate. There is very little data in the literature comparing benefits of one product versus the other [7, 8]. Antibacterial creams: mupirocin, Na-fusidate and bacitracin are also available for use in localized superficial skin infections [9]. Drawbacks of topical therapy include development of resistance, risk of irritant or allergic dermatitis (sensitization), and if used in high concentrations, these could cause burn injuries.

4. Invasive streptococcal infections: erysipelas and cellulitis

When skin infection results in erythematous (red in color), edematous (raised above the surface) and well demarcated (sharp boundary between involved and uninvolved skin) areas of involvement, it is referred to as **Erysipelas** (**Figure 2**). Erysipelas is characterized by marked edema in the skin, sometimes severe enough to cause skin blisters. While it could be seen at any age, it is more common in the very young and in older individuals. Classically described as occurring on the face, it can be seen in other parts of the body including the trunk and extremities. It is commonly associated with systemic symptoms like fever, chills and body ache, and blood cultures could be positive. Erysipelas is most commonly caused by *S. pyogenes* but could also be caused by other streptococci and less commonly by *S. aureus* [10]. Superficial skin culture should not be obtained, and causative organism can be established if blood cultures return positive. The diagnosis is usually clinical and it responds well to antibiotic therapy. However, in patients with uncontrolled diabetes or other immunocompromising conditions, the infection can spread deeper and the patient could develop sepsis and shock. Recurrences—especially on the extremities—are common in patients with underlying chronic lymphedema [11].

When streptococcal infection involves the skin as well as the subcutaneous tissue, it results in ill-defined areas of erythema that are rapidly spreading and this is called **Cellulitis.** The skin appears red with irregular spreading borders (**Figure 3**). The entry point for the infection is a break in the skin like a surgical wound or other skin trauma, underlying dermatoses like eczema and psoriasis or a fungal infection of the intertriginous areas like web spaces of the toes: "athlete's foot" (**Figure 4**). The area of the skin involved is tender to touch, and cellulitis is associated with systemic symptoms like fever, chills and body ache. Sometimes infection spreads along a lymphatic channel rather than the entire skin and this is called **streptococcal lymphangitis**

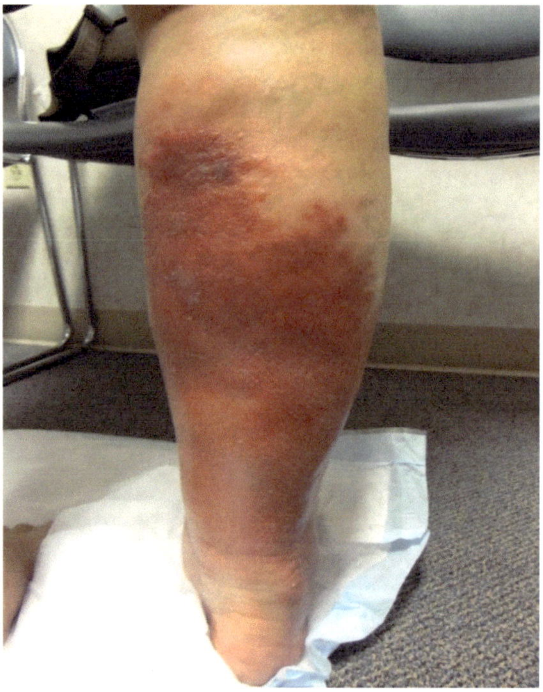

Figure 2.
Erysipelas with sharply-defined edematous red skin lesions.

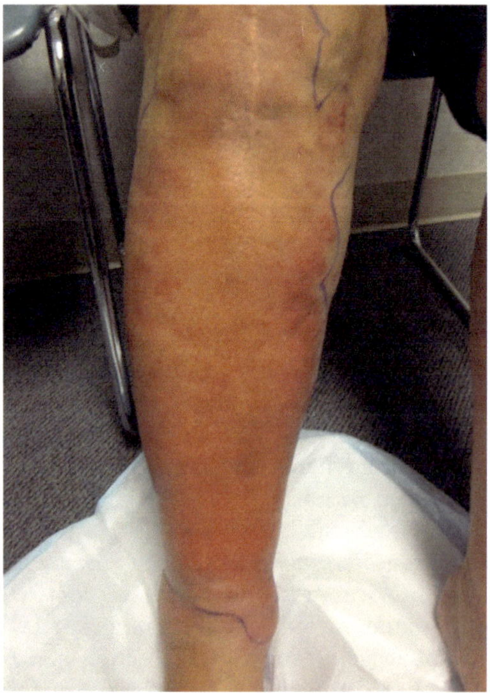

Figure 3.
Cellulitis with irregular and ill-defined borders.

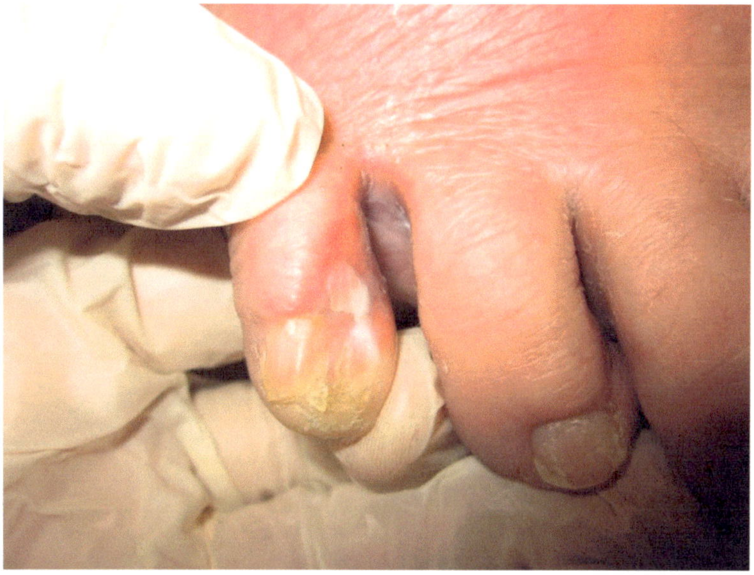

Figure 4.
Fungal infection in the webspace of the toes, also called "athlete's foot."

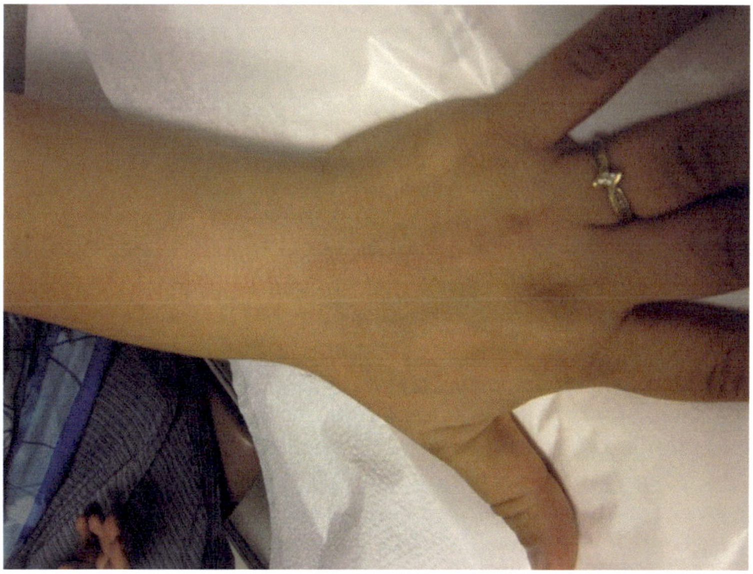

Figure 5.
Lymphangitic streaking of the upper extremity.

(**Figures 5** and **6**). Blood cultures are positive in around 10% of cases [12, 13] which include patients with more severe disease, older patients, patients with underlying liver cirrhosis [12] and diabetes [13]. The yield of blood cultures is higher if cultures are obtained at the time when the patient is experiencing fever and chills. Cellulitis responds very quickly to appropriate antibiotic therapy. As with erysipelas, recurrences are common in those with underlying risk factors, and left untreated, the infection can spread to deeper tissues and result in sepsis and shock.

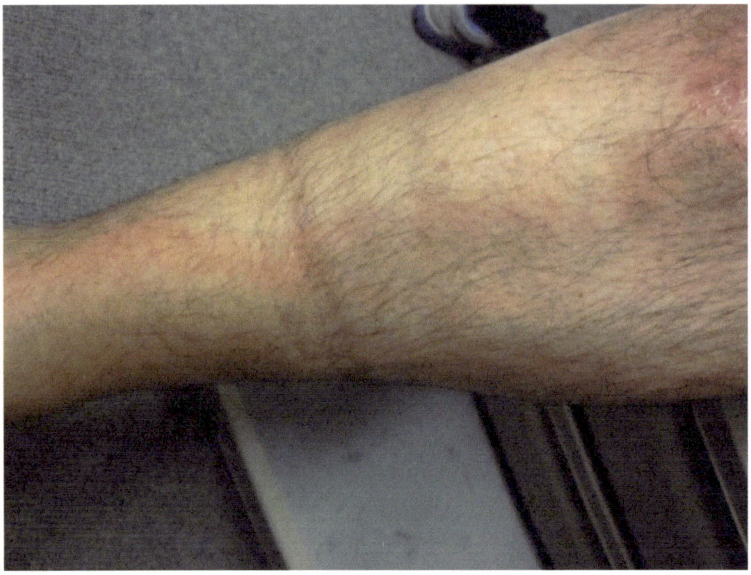

Figure 6.
Lymphangitic streaking (double) of the lower extremity.

In some patients there is an overlap between erysipelas and cellulitis and the clinical differences are not so clear. Importantly, management of both conditions is similar.

5. Treatment of cellulitis and erysipelas

Mild localized infections are treated with oral antibiotics, while more extensive infections or infections with systemic symptoms are treated with parenteral (intravenous) antibiotic therapy [14]. Patients with signs of sepsis: fever or hypothermia, tachycardia and hypotension, and patients with underlying conditions like uncontrolled diabetes, liver cirrhosis, severe peripheral vascular disease or severe lymphedema and patients with immunocompromising conditions like HIV, or patients on chemotherapy should be admitted to the hospital for antibiotics as well as aggressive management of the underlying conditions. Penicillins and β-lactams are considered the antibiotics of choice for treatment of streptococcal cellulitis. The addition of a second antibiotic like trimethoprim/sulfamethoxazole (TMP/SMX) or clindamycin has been shown to provide no additional benefit [6, 15–18]. Penicillins are available in the form of oral as well as intravenous preparations (**Table 1**). Extended spectrum penicillins: dicloxacillin, amoxicillin, ampicillin, oxacillin and nafcillin can be used if there is associated methicillin susceptible *S. aureus* (MSSA) infection. Cephalosporins are among the most commonly used β-lactams for the treatment of cellulitis. Different preparations are available both in the oral as well as the intravenous forms (**Table 2**). Physician preference and dosing convenience often define the choice of the antibiotic prescribed. Ceftaroline—one of the newest cephalosporins has excellent skin penetration and has activity against methicillin resistant *S. aureus* (MRSA) [19]. Patients who have an allergy to penicillin will require alternate agents. It should be noted here that there is increasing evidence in the literature

Name	Dosage	Comments
Oral agents		
Penicillin VK	250–500 mg, 4 times a day	
Dicloxacillin	250–500 mg, 4 times a day	Effective also against MSSA
Amoxicillin	500 mg, 3 times a day	Effective also against MSSA
Intravenous agents		
Penicillin G	2–4 million units, q 4–6 h	Also available as continuous infusion via pump
Ampicillin	2 g, q 4–6 h	Effective also against MSSA
Oxacillin, Nafcillin	1–2 g, q 4–6 h	Effective also against MSSA
Piperacillin-tazobactam*	4.5 g, q 8 h	Effective also against MSSA, *Pseudomona*, anaerobic bacteria

**Require dose adjustment in patients with kidney disease.*

Table 1.
Penicilins.

	Name	Dosage
Oral cephalosporins		
1st generation	cephalexin	500 mg, 4 time a day
2nd generation	cefaclor	500 mg, 3 times a day
	cefuroxime	500 mg, 2 times a day
3rd generation	cefpodoxime	200 mg, 2 times a day
Intravenous cephalosporins		
1st generation	cefazolin	1–2 g, q 8 h
3rd generation	ceftriaxone	1–2 g, q 24 h
5th generation	Ceftaroline	600 mg, q 12 h
Carbapenems (Intravenous)		
	Imipenem	0.5–1 g q 6 h
	Meropenem	1–2 g, q 8 h
	Ertapenem	1 g, q 24 h

Effective also against MSSA. Ceftaroline is also effective against MRSA.
All (except ceftriaxone) require dose adjustment in patients with kidney disease.

Table 2.
β-Lactam antibiotics used for streptococcal skin infections.

indicating patients who claim penicillin allergy may not have a true allergy and are able to tolerate β-lactams [20, 21]. TMP-SMX [22], doxycycline, linezolid, clindamycin and fluoroquinolones (**Table 3**) all have excellent skin penetration and may be used as alternate oral agents in patients with allergies to penicillin and β-lactams. Severe cellulitis in patients who have a true allergy to both penicillin and β-lactams is

Name	Drug class	Dose	Comments
Oral agents			
TMP/SMX* (160 mg/800 mg)	Sulphonamide	1–2 tabs, 2 times a day	Effective also against MSSA, MRSA
			Watch for rash, monitor cbc, creatinine
Doxycycline, Minocycline (100 mg)	Tetracycline derivative	1 tab, 2 times a day	Effective also against MSSA, MRSA
			Risk for sunburn, pill esophagitis
Linezolid (600 mg)	Oxazolidinone	1 tab, 2 times a day	Effective also against MSSA, MRSA
			Avoid co-administration with SSRI, MAO inhibitors
			Risk for cytopenias, neuropathy
			Excellent oral-parenteral bioavailability
Clindamycin (300 mg)	Lincosamide	300–450 mg, 4 times a day	Effective also against MSSA, MRSA
			Highest risk for CDiff infection
Ciprofloxacin, levofloxacin, moxifloxacin	Fluoroquinolone*	Different doses for different agents	Effective also against MSSA
			Risk for tendon injury, CNS side effects in the elderly, CDiff infection
Intravenous agents			Effective also against MSSA, MRSA
Vancomycin*	Glycopeptide	15–20 mg/kg q 12 h	Close monitoring of levels to avoid nephrotoxicity. Red-man syndrome if administered too fast
Daptomycin*	Cyclic lipopeptide	4–6 mg/kg q 24 h	Risk of rhabdomyolysis, Esosinophilic pneumonia
Linezolid	Oxazolidinone	600 mg q 12 h	Avoid co-administration with SSRI, MAO inhibitors
			Risk for cytopenias, neuropathy
Tigecycline	Tetracycline derivative (glycylcycline)	100 mg X 1, then 50 mg q 12 h	Effective also against anaerobes
			Risk for Nausea

**Require dose adjustment in patients with kidney disease.*

Table 3.
Non β-lactam antibiotics used for streptococcal skin infections.

treated with intravenous (IV) vancomycin. IV vancomycin requires close monitoring of levels to achieve optimized benefits while avoiding nephrotoxicity [23, 24], and often therapeutic levels are difficult to achieve in obese individuals [25]. Other alternatives to β-lactams are listed in **Table 3**. Daptomycin is a lipopeptide antibiotic that has excellent skin penetration [26, 27]. It has the advantage of once- a- day

Name	Drug class	Dose	Comments
Dalbavancin	Lipo-glycopeptide	Intravenous: 1.5 g single dose	One dose IV provides 2 weeks of therapy
Oritavancin	Lipo-glycopeptide	Intravenous: 1.2 g single dose	One dose IV provides 2 weeks of therapy
Delafloxacin	Fluoroquinolone	Intravenous: 300 mg q 12 h Oral: 450 mg twice a day	Allows transition from IV to oral. Risks as with other FQ
Omadacycline	Tetracycline derivative	Intravenous: 200 mg X 1, then 100 mg daily Oral: 450 mg once a day for 2 days, then 300 mg once a day	Allows transition from IV to oral. Gastrointestinal side effects. Effective also against anaerobes
Tedizolid	Oxazolidinone	Intravenous: 200 mg, q 24 h Oral: 200 mg once a day	Allows transition from IV to oral. Risk for cytopenias, neuropathy

Effective also against MSSA, MRSA.

Table 4.
Newer antibiotics approved for treatment of skin infections.

dosing, making daptomycin a convenient agent for outpatient antibiotic therapy (OPAT). Other antibiotics with excellent skin penetration include linezolid [28, 29] and tigecycline [27, 30]. Both these antibiotics are dosed twice a day and hence less convenient for use as OPAT. Tigecycline is only available in the parenteral form and is recommended for patients hospitalized with severe infections. Linezolid is available in both parenteral as well as oral formulations. IV linezolid is used when a patient is hospitalized with severe cellulitis, and treatment can be completed with oral formulation once the patient improves. There are a number of newer agents approved for the management of SSTIs including long acting lipo-glycopeptide agents oritavancin and dalbavancin, extended-spectrum fluoroquinolone delafloxacin, and the new tetracycline derivative omadacycline [28, 29]. Important comments regarding the advantages as well as the potential side effects of these antibiotics are listed in **Tables 3** and **4**.

6. Streptococcal infection of deeper tissues

When streptococcal infection spreads deep beyond the subcutaneous tissue, it can result in extensive necrosis (gangrene) of the overlying skin and inflammation and necrosis of underlying fascia **(Streptococcal Necrotizing Fasciitis)** and even muscle (**Streptococcal Myositis**). These infections are considered surgical emergencies.

Necrotizing Fasciitis (NF) is characterized by rapidly (within hours) spreading infection of the skin, subcutaneous tissue and fascia with associated symptoms of fever, prostration, hypotension and shock. It carries a high mortality [31]. It could start as a benign appearing skin wound that rapidly spreads both on the surface as well as into deeper tissues and the entire limb or body-part could be involved in a matter of a few hours. Skin changes include a rapid progression from mild erythema to a dusky appearance followed by ecchymosis, purpura, blisters and tissue

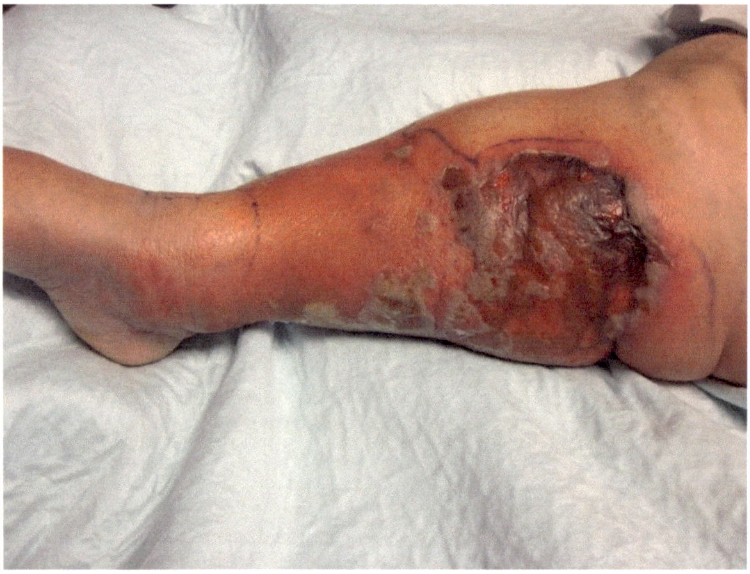

Figure 7.
Necrotizing fasciitis of the lower extremity.

necrosis—resulting in open wounds often discharging purulent or hemorrhagic fluid (**Figures** 7 and **8**). "Pain out of proportion to physical findings" is a characteristic sign of NF. In other words, there may be pain when palpating areas beyond the visible area of redness or in other cases even gentle palpation of involved area elicits excruciating pain. Some authorities divide NF into type I and type II. Type I is characterized by poly-microbial infection (involving both aerobic as well as anaerobic bacteria), while type II is characterized by mono-microbial infection of which

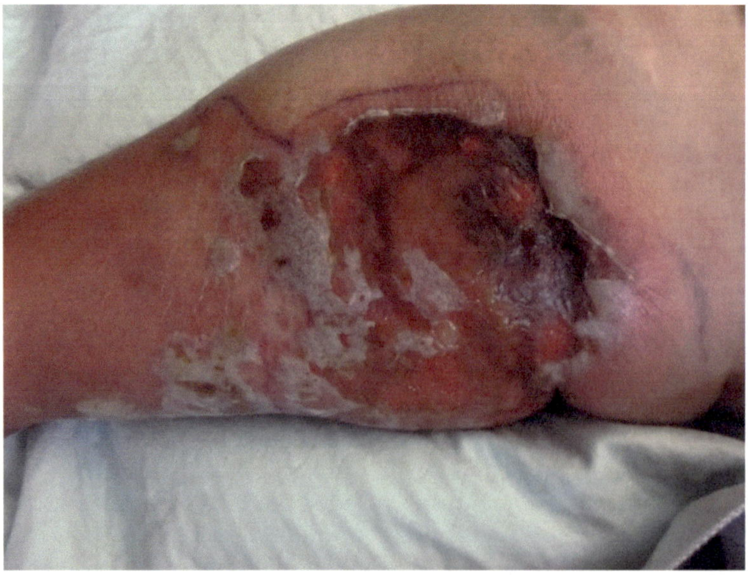

Figure 8.
Clinical photograph showing erythema, peeling skin, dusky hue and areas of necrosis.

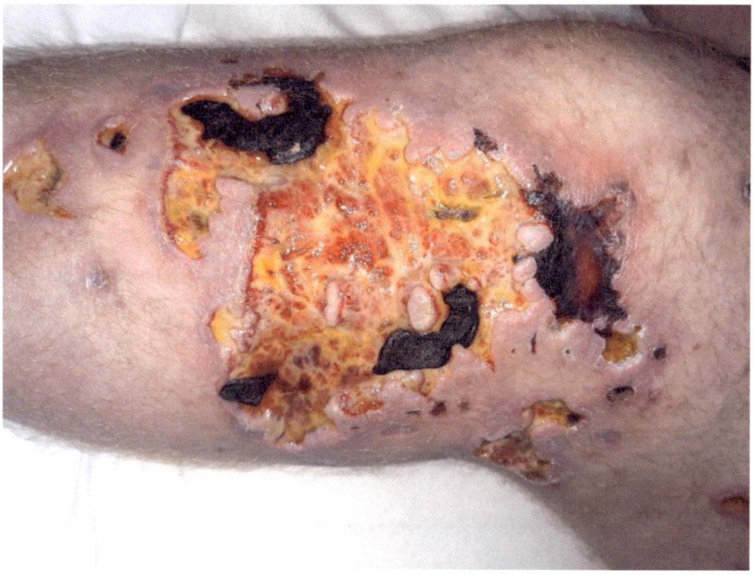

Figure 9.
Necrotic areas with skip lesions on leg of patient who is abusing self with injection drugs.

group A streptococcus is the most commonly implicated organism [32]. Mortality was found to be lower in *group A streptococcus*—associated NF (type II) compared to type I: 10% versus 20% in one large study [31]. NF may also be seen in persons who inject drugs. In these cases, multiple skip lesions are seen (**Figure 9**) and infection is usually poly-microbial. In addition to the skin lesions, the patient usually has systemic symptoms of sepsis including high fever, tachycardia, hypotension and may progress to have multi-organ failure. Streptococcal pyrogenic exotoxins

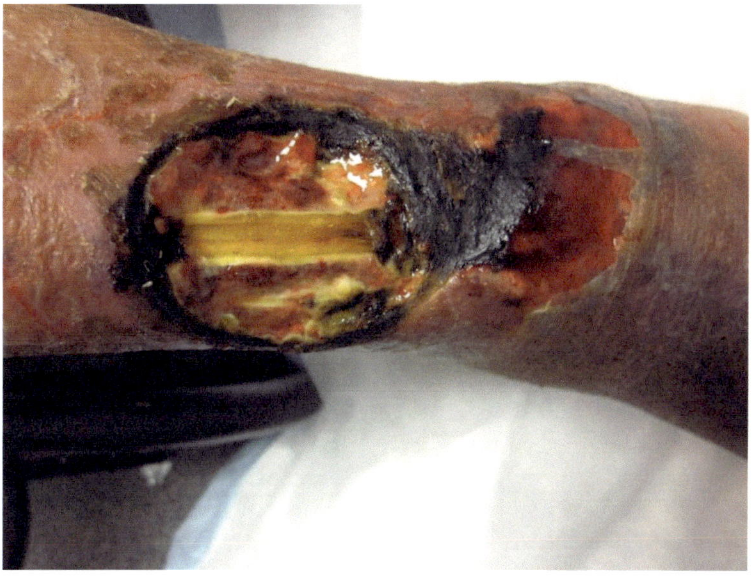

Figure 10.
Necrosis of skin, soft tissue and muscle with exposure of tendon.

(Spe) A, B and C are responsible for causing stimulation of a severe inflammatory cascade resulting in injury not only at the area of infection (local necrosis) but also to distant sites (lungs, kidneys, liver, central nervous system). Blood cultures are universally positive, and imaging of involved body-part (CT scan or MRI) will demonstrate edema and/or gas in the soft tissue planes and other changes consistent with this diagnosis [33].

When infection spreads beyond the fascial planes into the underlying muscles it is called myositis. **Streptococcal myositis** is often a complication of the overlying skin infection. Sometimes a deep tissue hematoma caused by blunt trauma [34] could get inoculated by the organism in a patient with bacteremia. This too is an emergency and requires rapid surgical intervention to relieve the pressure created by the severe inflammation in the muscle planes (**Figure 10**). Patients will also have systemic symptoms and signs of sepsis as seen in NF. There is often overlap of these two conditions in many patients.

7. Management of necrotizing fasciitis and streptococcal myositis

Patients need admission to the hospital often to the intensive care unit. They require management by a team of experts involving medical, surgical, infectious diseases and critical care specialties. They often present with septic shock and require pressors like epinephrine, norepinephrine and vasopressin to maintain adequate blood pressure in order to perfuse critical organs. Patients require broad spectrum antibiotic coverage, aggressive fluid resuscitation, as well as emergent aggressive debridement of the infected areas. Surgical removal of infected/necrotic tissue is essential in order to reduce bacterial burden and hence remove the source of toxins. Often patients require a second or even third visit to the operating room because of extensive tissue necrosis not amenable to removal in a single operation [14]. Operative tissue is sent for microbiology (cultures) to help determine the infectious agent and obtain an antibiotic sensitivity profile to help guide appropriate antibiotic choices. While awaiting the results of cultures, the antibiotics chosen should cover Gram-positive bacteria including *Streptococcus* and *S. aureus*, Gram-negative bacteria including drug-resistant bacteria like *Pseudomonas*, as well as anaerobic bacteria. Different combinations of antibiotics from **Tables 1–3** can be used. IV vancomycin (or IV daptomycin) plus cefepime (or fluoroquinolone) plus metronidazole, or IV vancomycin (or IV daptomycin) plus meropenem (or imipenem), or IV daptomycin plus piperacillin- tazobactam are some potential options for empiric therapy. Linezolid could be used in place of vancomycin and daptomycin in the above combinations. Vancomycin, daptomycin and linezolid provide Gram-positive coverage, cefepime and fluoroquinolones provide Gram-negative coverage. While metronidazole provides only anaerobic coverage, imipenem, meropenem and piperacillin-tazobactam provide Gram-negative as well as anaerobic coverage. Clindamycin is added in the initial critical stages of the infection on account of its antitoxin effect [14, 33]. If linezolid is used, additional clindamycin is not required because linezolid itself also has an antitoxin effect [33]. When culture results become available, antibiotics should be deescalated to target the organisms identified. Intravenous immunoglobulins (IVIG) is used at some centers as part of management of NF, however large studies have not shown a statistically significant benefit compared to those patients who did not receive IVIG [14, 33].

8. Toxic shock syndrome (TSS)

TSS is associated with a dramatic widespread skin rash and severe systemic symptoms. This condition is not due to direct inoculation of the skin with *Streptococcus*, but rather it is secondary to exotoxin [35] released by *Streptococcus* infection at a

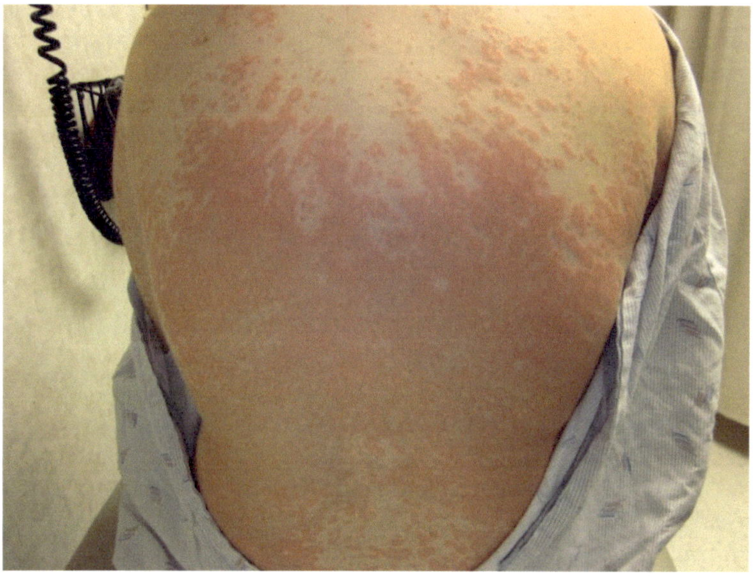

Figure 11.
Clinical photograph of sheet of erythema seen in acute phase of toxic shock syndrome.

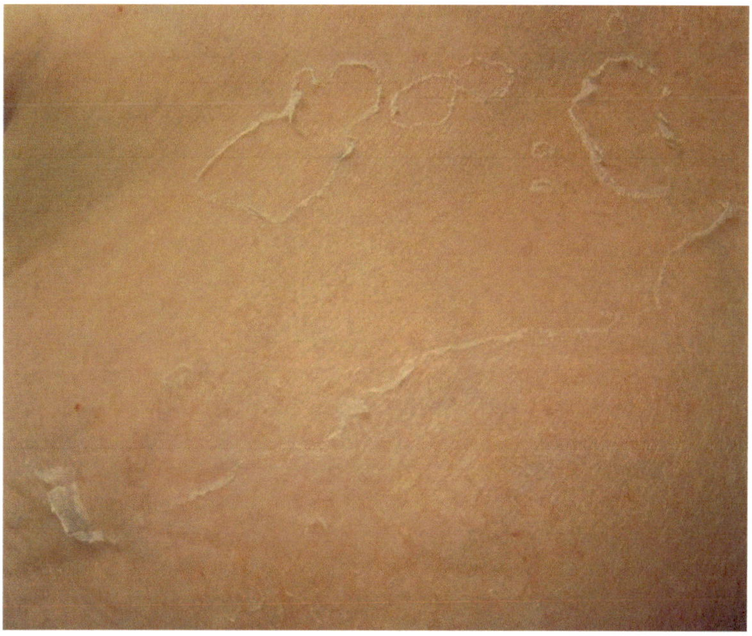

Figure 12.
Toxic shock syndrome with desquamation in the recovery phase.

distant site. Originally described in children with *S. aureus* infection, TSS is seen with *Streptococcus* and Clostridial infection in children as well as adults [36]. Patients present with widespread rash associated with fever, hypotension and multi-organ system involvement as a result of circulating streptococcal exotoxins A, B and C. The rash is described as sheets of erythema (**Figure 11**) involving the face, trunk as well as extremities, and it subsides with characteristic desquamation (**Figure 12**) when the patient recovers. A detailed examination is important to determine the source of infection: either retained foreign body like menstrual tampon or surgical sponge/ dressing material, necrotizing infection in a deep space, post-operative wound infection or peritonitis. Rarely, streptococcal pharyngitis is the primary event. The circulating toxins (super-antigens) are responsible for injury to internal organs—lungs, kidneys, liver [35] and the disease can be fatal in 40 to 60% cases of streptococcal TSS especially when there is delay in the diagnosis and hence delayed initiation of appropriate antibiotics. Blood cultures may be positive, as are cultures from an identified focus of infection.

9. Management of TSS

As with other severe streptococcal infection, patients with TSS require admission to the hospital. If they are hypotensive or experience multi-organ failure, management is in the intensive care unit where patients are treated with aggressive fluid resuscitation, broad antibiotic therapy (choices similar to that as described for management of necrotizing fasciitis) and pressor support. Surgery may be required if a deep focus of infection is identified. Rarely patients do not respond to standard therapy and may require intravenous immunoglobulins (IVIG) [36].

10. Discussion on general principles of systemic antibiotic therapy

Streptococcal SSTIs respond very well to antibiotic therapy. A wide range of antibiotics with excellent skin penetration are now available as noted in **Tables 1–4**. All antibiotics carry the potential for side effects like allergic reactions and gastrointestinal disturbances. There are some side effects that are unique to certain antibiotics and patients need to be monitored for these toxicities. For example: β-lactam antibiotics have the potential for hepatotoxicity, vancomycin is associated with nephrotoxicity, daptomycin can cause rhabdomyolysis and eosinophilic pneumonitis and clindamycin is one of the most common antibiotics associated with *Clostridioides difficile* (*C. Diff*) infection. In addition, inappropriate use of broad-spectrum antibiotics—and even prolonged use of narrow spectrum antibiotics—can result in collateral damage (destruction of protective normal bacterial flora of the skin and the gastrointestinal tract) and cause antibiotic-associated diarrhea and *C. Diff* infection [37, 38]. Indiscriminate use of broad-spectrum antibiotics has also contributed to the development of multidrug-resistant pathogens [39]. Therefore, judicious use of antibiotics is very important to reduce the risk of these complications. Streptococcal infections should be treated with narrow spectrum antibiotics like penicillin and β-lactams. When streptococcal cellulitis or erysipelas does not seem to be responding adequately within the first 2–3 days of β-lactam therapy, antibiotics with additional coverage against MRSA will need to be used.

11. Specific points regarding treatment of SSTIs

1. Mild infections should be treated with oral antibiotics.

2. Severe infections (severe local skin infection with systemic symptoms like fever, tachycardia, hypotension or leukocytosis and bacteremia, or more extensive skin infections even without systemic symptoms) will require parenteral therapy, with step-down to oral therapy as the patient improves [40]. Antibiotics like the floroquinolones: ciprofloxacin, levofloxacin, delafloxacin [41, 42], moxifloxacin [43], the oxazolidinones: linezolid, tedizolid and the new tetracycline: omadacycline [44] have excellent oral bioavailability and allow early conversion from intravenous to oral therapy.

3. In the most serious cases: sepsis, septic shock, necrotizing fasciitis, myositis, toxic shock syndrome: broad-spectrum antibiotics are required initially (most often with more than one antimicrobial agent) to cover *Streptococcus*, *S. aureus* including MRSA as well as gram-negative and anaerobic bacteria. "De-escalation" can be achieved once microbiology data (blood cultures, deep tissue and intra-operative cultures) are available to guide the final antibiotic choice targeting the bacteria identified.

4. Duration of antibiotics: This depends on the severity of the infection as well as the clinical response to therapy. Mild infections or even severe infections in an otherwise healthy host that respond rapidly to antibiotics could be treated for as short as 5 days [14, 45, 46]. More severe infections or infections with a delayed response to therapy may need longer courses like 7, 10 or 14 days, depending upon the clinical picture. Shorter courses may be possible with some of the newer antibiotics including single dose antibiotics like dalbavancin [47] and oritavancin [28]. Relapses are found to be more common in patients with shorter courses of therapy [45]. Patients with bacteremia are usually treated for 14 days.

5. Dose adjustments: Antibiotics are cleared by the liver or kidney and hence dosage needs to be reduced in patients with liver or kidney disease in order to avoid toxicity. Conversely, patients who are obese require a higher dose of the antibiotic to achieve therapeutic levels in the skin [25, 48].

6. Suppressive therapy is attempted for patients with multiple recurrences [45, 49, 50]. Oral penicillin twice daily showed a 70–80% reduction in episodes—but recurrences occurred after discontinuation of prophylaxis. Treatment of underlying factors like athlete's foot, chronic lymphedema, peripheral vascular disease and uncontrolled diabetes is also very important in the prevention of recurrences [11, 44, 45, 51].

12. Conclusions

Streptococcal skin infections cause significant morbidity all over the world, and severe infections like necrotizing fasciitis and toxic shock syndrome can be fatal. There is a wide spectrum of manifestations of skin infections ranging from mild superficial disease to deep necrotic and life-threatening infections. Skin infection is one of the most common reasons for prescriptions of antibiotics in the community as well as in hospitalized patients. Some of the most commonly used antibiotics have excellent skin penetration and hence the armamentarium to treat skin infections is quite large. Over the last few years there have been multiple new antibiotics approved for the treatment of skin infections and these should be reserved for treatment of severe infections not responding to the common antibiotics and for infections with multi-drug-resistant organisms. A thorough understanding of the different types of skin infections, as well as a detailed knowledge of the different antibiotics are essential for the early diagnosis and selection of the most appropriate antibiotic for the management of simple as well as complex skin infections.

Author details

Alwyn Rapose
University of Massachusetts Medical School, Reliant Medical Group, Worcester, Massachusetts, USA

*Address all correspondence to: Alwyn.rapose@reliantmedicalgroup.org

References

[1] Sims Sanyahumbi A, Colquhoun S, Wyber R, et al. Global disease burden of Group A *Streptococcus*. In: Ferretti JJ, Stevens DL, Fischetti VA, editors. *Streptococcus pyogenes*: Basic Biology to Clinical Manifestations. Oklahoma City (OK), USA: University of Oklahoma Health Sciences Center; 2016

[2] https://wwwnc.cdc.gov/eid/article/15/9/08-1228_article [Accessed: November 15, 2021]

[3] https://wwwnc.cdc.gov/eid/article/27/2/20-1945_article [Accessed: November 15, 2021]

[4] Norris AH, Shrestha NK, Allison GM, et al. 2018 Infectious Diseases Society of America Clinical Practice Guideline for the Management of Outpatient Parenteral Antimicrobial Therapy. Clinical Infectious Diseases. 2019;**68**(1):e1-e35

[5] Keyloun KR, Weber DJ, Gardstein BM, et al. Economic burden of hospital admissions for patients with acute bacterial skin and skin structure infections in the United States. Hospital Practice. 2018;**46**(5):278-286

[6] Jenkins TC, Sabel AL, Sarcone EE, et al. Skin and soft-tissue infections requiring hospitalization at an academic medical center: Opportunities for antimicrobial stewardship. Clinical Infectious Diseases. 2010;**51**(8):895-903

[7] Dumville JC, Lipsky BA, Hoey C, et al. Topical antimicrobial agents for treating foot ulcers in people with diabetes. Cochrane Database of Systematic Reviews. 2017;**6**(6):CD011038

[8] Delgado-Enciso I, Madrigal-Perez VM, Lara-Esqueda A, et al. Topical 5% potassium permanganate solution accelerates the healing process in chronic diabetic foot ulcers. Biomedical Reports. 2018;**8**(2):156-159

[9] Williamson DA, Carter GP, Howden BP. Current and emerging topical antibacterials and antiseptics: Agents, action, and resistance patterns. Clinical Microbiology Reviews. 2017;**30**(3):827-860

[10] Eriksson B, Jorup-Ronstrom C, Karkkonen K, et al. Erysipelas: Clinical and bacteriologic spectrum and serological aspects. Clinical Infectious Diseases. 1996;**23**(5):1091-1098

[11] Inghammar M, Rasmussen M, Linder A. Recurrent erysipelas-risk factors and clinical presentation. BMC Infectious Diseases. 2014;**14**(1):270-275

[12] Lee CY, Kunin CM, Chang C, et al. Development of a prediction model for bacteremia in hospitalized adults with cellulitis to aid in the efficient use of blood cultures: A retrospective cohort study. BMC Infectious Diseases. 2016;**16**(1):581

[13] Lasa JS, Fernández Recalde ML, Finn BC, et al. Bacteremia in patients hospitalized with cellulitis. Medicina (B Aires). 2012;**72**(4):298-304

[14] Stevens DL, Bisno AL, Chambers HF, et al. Infectious Diseases Society of America Practice guidelines for the diagnosis and management of skin and soft tissue infections: 2014 update by the Infectious Diseases Society of America. Clinical Infectious Diseases. 2014;**59**:e10-e52

[15] Madaras-Kelly KJ, Remington RE, Oliphant CM, et al. Efficacy of oral

beta-lactam versus non-beta-lactam treatment of uncomplicated cellulitis. The American Journal of Medicine. 2008;**121**(5):419-425

[16] Jeng A, Beheshti M, Li J, et al. The role of beta-hemolytic streptococci in causing diffuse, nonculturable cellulitis: A prospective investigation. Medicine (Baltimore). 2010;**89**(4):217-226

[17] Pallin DJ, Binder WD, Allen MB, et al. Clinical trial: Comparative effectiveness of cephalexin plus trimethoprim-sulfamethoxazole versus cephalexin alone for treatment of uncomplicated cellulitis: A randomized controlled trial. Clinical Infectious Diseases. 2013;**56**(12):1754-1762

[18] Brindle R, Williams OM, Davies P, et al. Adjunctive clindamycin for cellulitis: A clinical trial comparing flucloxacillin with or without clindamycin for the treatment of limb cellulitis. BMJ Open. 2017;**7**(3):e013260

[19] Santos PD, Davis A, Jandourek A, et al. Ceftaroline fosamil and treatment of acute bacterial skin and skin structure infections: CAPTURE study experience. Chemotherapy. 2013;**25**(6):341-346

[20] Blumenthal KG, Peter JG, Trubiano JA, et al. Antibiotic allergy. Lancet. 2019;**393**(10167):183-198

[21] Staicu ML, Vyles D, Shenoy ES, et al. Penicillin allergy delabeling: A multidisciplinary opportunity. The Journal of Allergy and Clinical Immunology. 2020;**8**(9):2858-2868

[22] Bowen AC, Carapetis JR, Currie BJ, et al. Sulfamethoxazole-Trimethoprim (Cotrimoxazole) for skin and soft tissue infections including impetigo, cellulitis, and abscess. Open Forum Infectious Diseases. 2017;**4**(4):ofx232

[23] Rybak MJ, Le J, Lodise TP, et al. Therapeutic monitoring of vancomycin for serious methicillin-resistant *Staphylococcus aureus* infections: A revised consensus guideline and review by the American Society of Health-System Pharmacists, the Infectious Diseases Society of America, the Pediatric Infectious Diseases Society, and the Society of Infectious Diseases Pharmacists. American Journal of Health-System Pharmacy. 2020;**77**(11):835-864

[24] Jorgensen SCJ, Murray KP, Lagnf AM, et al. A multicenter evaluation of vancomycin-associated acute kidney injury in hospitalized patients with acute bacterial skin and skin structure infections. Infectious Disease and Therapy. 2020;**9**(1):89-106

[25] Smit C, Wasmann RE, Goulooze SC, et al. Population pharmacokinetics of vancomycin in obesity: Finding the optimal dose for (morbidly) obese individuals. British Journal of Clinical Pharmacology. 2020;**86**(2):303-317

[26] Sauermann R, Rothenburger M, Graninger W, et al. Daptomycin: A review 4 years after first approval. Pharmacology. 2008;**81**(2):79-91

[27] Eckmann C, Dryden M. Treatment of complicated skin and soft-tissue infections caused by resistant bacteria: Value of linezolid, tigecycline, daptomycin and vancomycin. European Journal of Medical Research. 2010;**15**(12):554-563

[28] Golan Y. Current treatment options for acute skin and skin-structure infections. Clinical Infectious Diseases. 2019;**68**(Suppl. 3):S206-S212

[29] Crotty MP, Krekel T, Burnham CA, et al. New gram-positive agents: The next generation of oxazolidinones and

lipoglycopeptides. Journal of Clinical Microbiology. 2016;**54**(9):2225-2232

[30] Grolman DC. Therapeutic applications of tigecycline in the management of complicated skin and skin structure infections. International Journal of Infectious Diseases. 2007;**11**(Suppl. 1):S7-S15

[31] Bruun T, Rath E, Madsen MB, et al. Risk factors and predictors of mortality in streptococcal necrotizing soft-tissue infections: A multicenter prospective study. INFECT Study Group. Clinical Infectious Diseases. 2021;**72**(2):293-300

[32] Kiat HJ, En Natalie YH, Fatimah LJ. Necrotizing fasciitis: How reliable are the cutaneous signs? Journal of Emergencies, Trauma and Shock. 2017;**10**(4):205-210

[33] Bonne SL, Kadri SS. Evaluation and management of necrotizing soft tissue infections. Infectious Disease Clinics of North America. 2017;**31**(3):497-511

[34] Nuwayhid ZB, Aronoff DM, Mulla ZD. Blunt trauma as a risk factor for group A streptococcal necrotizing fasciitis. Annals of Epidemiology. 2007;**17**(11):878-881

[35] Emgård J, Bergsten H, McCormick JK, et al. MAIT cells are major contributors to the cytokine response in group A streptococcal toxic shock syndrome. Proceedings of the National Academy of Sciences of the United States of America. 2019;**116**(51):25923-25931

[36] Rapose A. Toxic Shock Syndrome. In: Conn's Current Therapy. Philadelphia (PA), USA: Elsevier Health Sciences; 2021. pp. 666-668

[37] Brown KA, Khanafer N, Daneman N, et al. Meta-analysis of antibiotics and the risk of community-associated Clostridium difficile infection. Antimicrobial Agents and Chemotherapy. 2013;**57**(5):2326-2332

[38] Webb BJ, Subramanian A, Lopansri B, et al. Antibiotic exposure and risk for hospital-associated Clostridioides difficile infection. Antimicrobial Agents and Chemotherapy. 2020;**64**(4): e02169-e02119

[39] Moghnieh R, Estaitieh N, Mugharbil A, et al. Third generation cephalosporin resistant Enterobacteriaceae and multidrug resistant gram-negative bacteria causing bacteremia in febrile neutropenia adult cancer patients in Lebanon, broad spectrum antibiotics use as a major risk factor, and correlation with poor prognosis. Frontiers in Cellular and Infection Microbiology. 2015;**12**(5):11

[40] Nathwani D, Dryden M, Garau J. Early clinical assessment of response to treatment of skin and soft-tissue infections: How can it help clinicians? Perspectives from Europe. International Journal of Antimicrobial Agents. 2016;**48**(2):127-136

[41] O'Riordan W, McManus A, Teras J, et al. A comparison of the efficacy and safety of intravenous followed by oral delafloxacin with vancomycin plus aztreonam for the treatment of acute bacterial skin and skin structure infections: A phase 3, Multinational, Double-Blind, Randomized Study. PROCEED Study Group. Clinical Infectious Diseases. 2018;**67**(5):657-666

[42] Kingsley J, Mehra P, Lawrence LE, et al. A randomized, double-blind, Phase 2 study to evaluate subjective and objective outcomes in patients with acute bacterial skin and skin structure infections treated with delafloxacin, linezolid or vancomycin. The Journal of Antimicrobial Chemotherapy. 2016;**71**(3):821-829

[43] Gyssens IC, Dryden M, Kujath P, et al. A randomized trial of the efficacy and safety of sequential intravenous/oral moxifloxacin monotherapy versus intravenous piperacillin/tazobactam followed by oral amoxicillin/clavulanate for complicated skin and skin structure infections. The Journal of Antimicrobial Chemotherapy. 2011;**66**(11):2632-2642

[44] Abrahamian FM, Sakoulas G, Tzanis E, et al. Omadacycline for acute bacterial skin and skin structure infections. Clinical Infectious Diseases. 2019;**69**(Suppl. 1):S23-S32

[45] Cranendonk DR, Opmeer BC, van Agtmael MA, et al. Antibiotic treatment for 6 days versus 12 days in patients with severe cellulitis: A multicentre randomized, double-blind, placebo-controlled, non-inferiority trial. Clinical Microbiology and Infection. 2020;**26**(5):606-612

[46] Morris AD. Cellulitis and erysipelas. BMJ Clinical Evidence. 2008;**2008**:1708

[47] Bennett JW, Lewis JS, Ellis MW. Dalbavancin in the treatment of complicated skin and soft-tissue infections: A review. Therapeutics and Clinical Risk Management. 2008;**4**(1):31-40

[48] Grupper M, Nicolau DP. Obesity and skin and soft tissue infections: How to optimize antimicrobial usage for prevention and treatment? Current Opinion in Infectious Diseases. 2017;**30**(2):180-191

[49] Thomas KS, Crook AM, Nunn AJ, et al. Penicillin to prevent recurrent leg cellulitis. The New England Journal of Medicine. 2013;**368**(18):1695-1703

[50] Dalal A, Eskin-Schwartz M, Mimouni D, et al. Interventions for the prevention of recurrent erysipelas and cellulitis. Cochrane Database of Systematic Reviews. 2017;**6**(6):CD009758

[51] Wilcox M, Yan JL, Gonzalez PL, et al. Impact of underlying comorbidities on outcomes of patients treated with Ceftaroline Fosamil for complicated skin and soft tissue infections: Pooled results from three phase III Randomized Clinical Trials. Infectious Disease and Therapy. 2022;**11**(1):217-230

Section 2

Fungal Infectious Diseases

Chapter 3

Talaromyces marneffei Infection: Virulence Factors and Rapid Diagnostics

Sirida Youngchim

Abstract

Talaromyces (*Penicillium*) *marneffei* is a thermally dimorphic fungus that causes talaromycosis, and the pathogen is found throughout tropical and subtropical Asia. *T. marneffei* has specifically emerged as an opportunistic fungal pathogen in individuals with advanced HIV disease and, to a lesser extent, other immunocompromised conditions, but more recently talaromycosis is increasingly described in immunocompetent people. Due to the high mortality rate of up to 50%, understanding *T. marneffei* interactions with host immune responses and diagnostic modalities is vital to the development of strategies to reduce morbidity and mortality. In this chapter, we describe *T. marneffei* virulence factors that enhance the fungus' capacity for survival and growth in the host to lead to disease. We also discuss approaches for early diagnosis, which are essential to reduce the mortality rate in talaromycosis. Talaromycosis remains a neglected disease, but advances in our understanding of host-pathogen dynamics as well as the ongoing development of new diagnostic approaches are poised to enhance our capacity to combat this disease.

Keywords: *Talaromyces* (*Penicillium*) *marneffei*, dimorphic fungus, endemic mycoses, virulence factors, rapid diagnosis

1. Introduction

Talaromyces (*Penicillium*) *marneffei* is a thermally dimorphic fungus endemic in the tropical and subtropical regions of Asia (**Figure 1**) [1, 2]. It is by far the species that most commonly causes human illness in immunocompromised patients, especially those with AIDS over the last three decades, especially in endemic areas of Southeast Asia (Thailand, Vietnam, Myanmar), East Asia (southern mainland China, Hong Kong, and Taiwan area), and north-eastern India, resulting in a rapid increase in incidence [2, 3]. Talaromycosis is not only recognized in endemic areas, but it is also increasingly being recorded in travelers from non-endemic areas such as Australia, Belgium, France, Germany, Japan, the Netherlands, Oman, Sweden, Switzerland, Togo, the United Kingdom, and the United States [4–10]. Fever, weight loss, anemia, lymphadenopathy, hepatosplenomegaly, respiratory symptoms, and skin lesions were all common clinical manifestations of *T. marneffei*

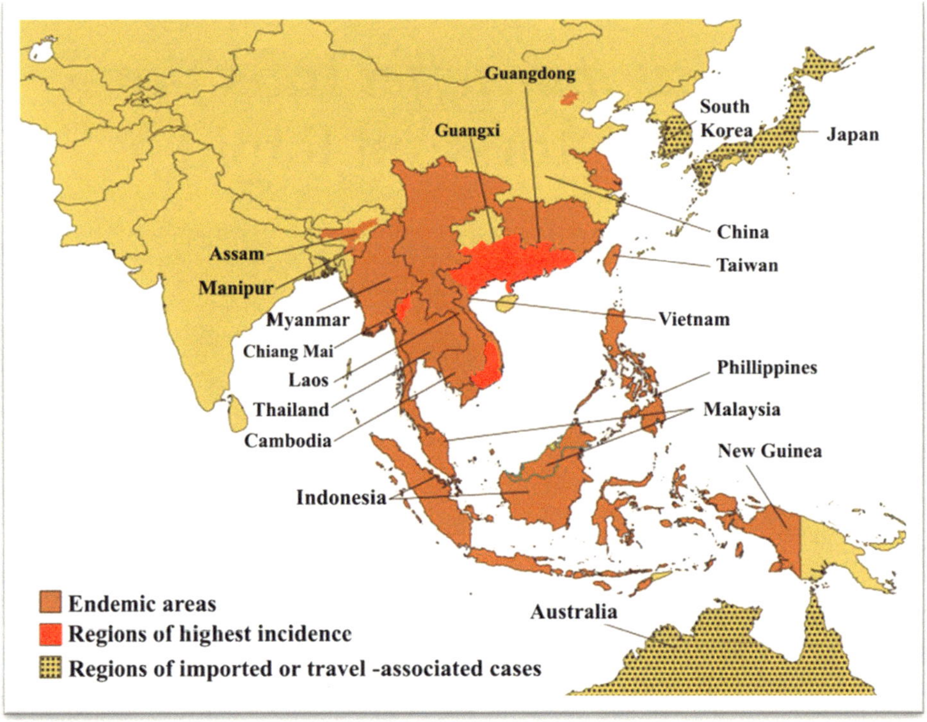

Figure 1.
Geographic distribution of talaromycosis.

infection. Furthermore, amphotericin B, itraconazole, and voriconazole were the most often used first-line treatments, either alone or in combination with other drugs. The majority of patients die if they are not treated.

Since 1994, talaromycosis is the fourth most general opportunistic infection, after tuberculosis, pneumocystis, and cryptococcosis in AIDS patients in Thailand [11, 12]. Currently, the number of *T. marneffei* infections has declined in the last few years because of a decreased incidence of HIV and widespread accessibility of antiretroviral therapy [13]. Talaromycosis is not limited to people living with HIV. It is becoming more common in non-HIV-infected people who have other immunosuppressive conditions, such as primary immunodeficiency, autoimmune diseases, cancer, and solid organ and bone marrow transplants [14]. Common clinical manifestations of infection caused by *T. marneffei* included fever, weight loss, anemia, lymphadenopathy, hepatosplenomegaly, respiratory signs, and skin lesions. Due to increased migration and global travel, talaromycosis is becoming more common outside of endemic areas [4]. Although most people with talaromycosis are immunocompromised, healthy people can be affected as well, although rarely [15]. Patients with advanced HIV disease (CD4 cell counts <100 cells/m^3) are at high risk; they typically occur with disseminated disease affecting the lungs, liver, spleen, gastrointestinal system, bloodstream, skin, and bone marrow [15]. Individuals without HIV are less likely than individuals with HIV to have skin lesions and positive blood cultures. As a result, as compared to HIV-positive persons, diagnosis is delayed (180 days vs. 45 days) and death is greater (29% vs. 21%) [16]. **Table 1** summarizes the laboratory findings and clinical prognosis of talaromycosis in patients with and without HIV infection.

Variable criteria	HIV-infected related	HIV-infected unrelated	Reference
Positive blood culture (%)	76.7	47.1	[17]
White blood cells (x 10^3cells/mm^3)	4.1	15.6	
CD4 (%)	3	30	
Lymphocytes (%)	11.8	16.4	[16]
Neutrophils (%)	81.2	75.2	
Skin lesions (%)	53.4	31.6	[16]
Diagnosis delayed (days)	45	180	[17]
Medium treatment duration (days)	84	180	[17]
Death (%)	21	29	[17]

Table 1.
The laboratory characteristics and clinical prognosis of talaromycosis in individuals with and without HIV infection.

Talaromycosis can affect both immunocompetent and immunocompromised patients, and the disease can be localized or systemic [18].

The ecology and route of transmission of *T. marneffei* infection are unknown. The organism has been isolated from the internal organs of four species of bamboo rats (*Rhizomys sinensis*, *R. pruinosus*, *R. sumatranensis*, and the reddish-brown subspecies of *Cannomys badius*) as well as the soil environment in which they dwell [19, 20]. A recent occupational history or other exposures to fine soil dust during the rainy season were determined to be the most important risk factors for illness. Contact with or consumption of bamboo rats do not appear to be significant risk factors for *T. marneffei* infection [21].

2. Culture and morphological characteristics

2.1 Macroscopic and microscopic appearances

T. marneffei is classified as a thermally dimorphic fungus which grows as a saprophytic mold. The fungus produces abundant conidia at 25°C and converts to yeast cells at 37°C. Mycelial colonies grow relatively quickly on Potato dextrose agar (PDA) at 25°C, as do other *Penicillium* species, and appear as flat, powdery white colonies. With continued culture, the periphery of the colony becomes more rugose, with radial folds. The color of the fungal colony changes from white to light brown and becomes light green after 10 days of culture. The colony produces diffusible red pigments into the agar and the underside of the colony (**Figure 2A**). This pigment production is one of the most characteristic features of *T. marneffei*. The microscopic examination of the mycelia phase reveals typical morphology of *Penicillium* or *Talaromyces* species. The microscopic examination of the mycelial form of *T. marneffei* is recognized as dense brush-like, spore-bearing structures (**Figure 2B**). The conidiophores can be simple or branched structures with clusters of flask-shaped phialides at the ends. The conidiophores are hyaline, smooth-walled and have terminal verticils of 3 to 5 metulae, each with 3 to 7 phialides [1].

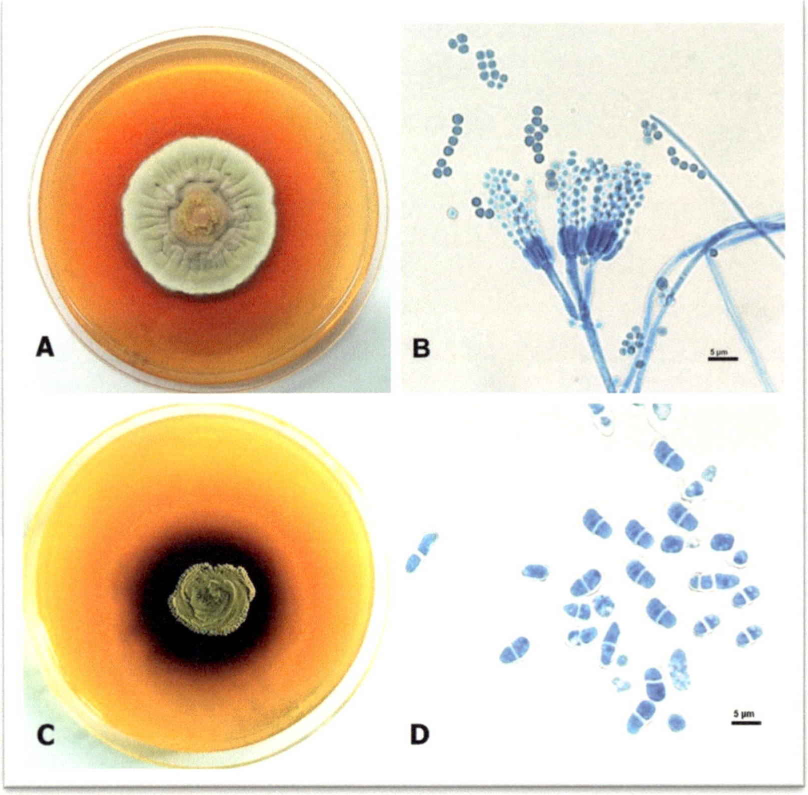

Figure 2.
Thermal dimorphism of Talaromyces marneffei: (A) at 25°C, T. marneffei was grown on PDA as a mold, producing greenish-yellow to yellow conidia and secreting a distinctive diffusible red pigment; (B) conidiophores have phialides and conidia chains that resemble those of Penicillium species; (C) at 37°C, T. marneffei grows as a yeast with a dark-brown colony on BHI agar, producing brown pigment; (D) yeast cells are divided by fission rather than budding. Bars, 5 µm.

At 37°C on Brain heart infusion (BHI) agar, *T. marneffei* can convert to yeast phase growth. Macroscopically, yeast-like colonies appear cebriform, convoluted, or smooth. Colonies are glabrous and beige-colored and take up to 10–14 days to exhibit full growth. Pigment production is both decreased and altered; the pigment released from *T. marneffei* yeast cultures appears closer to brown in color in comparison with the red pigment released from *T. marneffei* mycelial cultures (**Figure 2C**). Microscopically, yeast cells of *T. marneffei* are spherical to ellipsoidal yeast like cells separating by single septum, measuring 2–3 to 2–6 µm (**Figure 2D**) [22].

3. Virulence attributes of *T. marneffei*

It is generally believed that inhalation of *T. marneffei* conidia is the likely route for infection, in line with the mode of infection for other molds such as *Aspergillus fumigatus* [23, 24] and *Histoplasma capsulatum* [25]. Indeed, *T. marneffei* conidia are presumably small enough (2 µm in diameter) to reach the alveoli of the lung and then are subsequently phagocytized by pulmonary histiocytes. *T. marneffei*, however, is able to live and develop inside this hostile intracellular environment rather than being killed

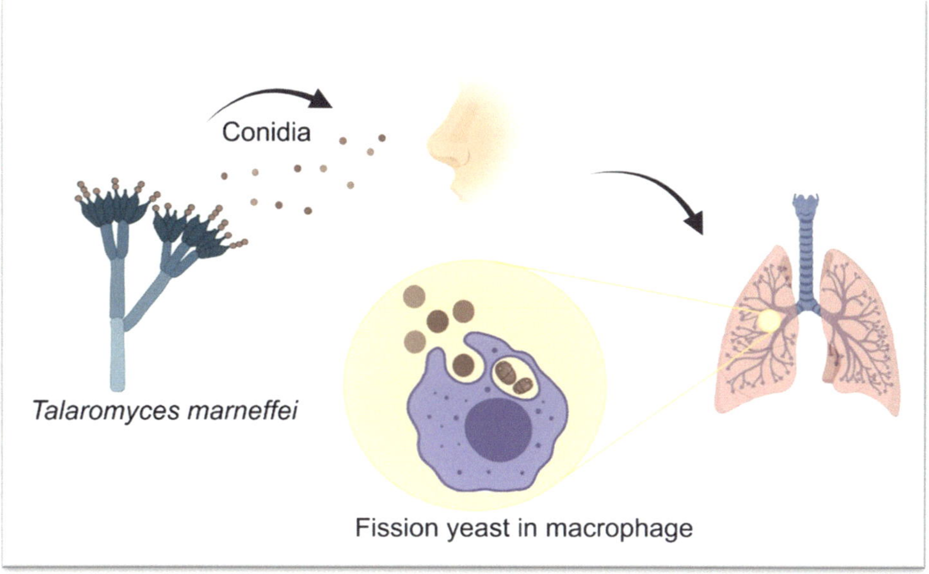

Figure 3.
A depiction of the acquisition process of mycelial T. marneffei from the environment to the lung with the transformation to fission yeast in macrophage after deposition in alveoli.

by the action of these immune cells (**Figure 3**). Then, *T. marneffei* can be disseminated throughout the body once established within the phagocyte and cause systemic infection if the host's immunological state is impaired. Indeed, a better knowledge of how the virulence pathways of *T. marneffei* interact with the immunological response of the host has helped us in redefining the pathogenesis of this fungus.

3.1 Adherence to host tissues

Adherence to host tissues by *T. marneffei* conidia may play an extremely important role in the establishment of talaromycosis. Although the infective propagule and route of entry have not been definitively confirmed, inhalation of fungal conidia is likely to be the proposed route of infection [1]. Indeed, *T. marneffei* conidia are tiny enough (2 μm in diameter) to reach the lung's alveoli, and the identify of a potential conidial laminin/fibronectin receptor in *T. marneffei* suggests a plausible mode of conidia attachment to the pulmonary epithelium [26, 27]. *T. marneffei* also bind extracellular matrix (ECM)-associated glycosaminoglycans, chondroitin sulfate B, heparin, and highly sulfated chitosan CP-3, which are major constituents of many tissues particularly the basal lamina [28]. These ECM may become exposed in the lung as a result of tissue damage facilitating conidia adhesion to the bronchoalveolar epithelium. Nonetheless, this hypothesis has yet to be confirmed in animal models. Following that, *T. marneffei* glyceraldehyde-3-phosphate dehydrogenase (GAPDH) was identified and acted as an adherence protein to facilitate conidia attachment to the host's bronchoalveolar epithelium suggesting that this protein may play an important role in the establishment of disease [29]. Indeed, knowledge of the adherence mechanisms in *T. marneffei* is still limited. The development of proteomic tools and the availability of genomic data will be of great importance to elucidate the mechanisms of the host-fungus interplay, and particularly of its adherence to the host tissues.

3.2 Dimorphic switching

Fungal morphogenesis appears to be a critical factor in infection establishment. Indeed, dimorphic switching between mycelial and yeast phases is regarded to be a significant virulence component in dimorphic pathogenic fungi including *H. capsulatum*, *Coccidioides immitis, Paracoccidioides brasiliensis*, *Blastomyces dermatitis*, and *T. marneffei* [30]. Conversion to the yeast form may provide protection against killing by neutrophils, monocytes, and macrophages. Thermal dimorphism of *T. marneffei* is essential for survival in host cells that are responsible for the host temperature change. During the past decade, significant progress has been made in the understanding of the phase transition to yeast forms. *T. marneffei* has the ability to change morphology from hyphal mold in the environment to pathogenic yeast cells once conidia are inhaled into the lung of a mammalian host. Within the human host, *T. marneffei* conidia are engulfed and destroyed by the host's phagocytes, particularly alveolar macrophages. After internalized conidia, *T. marneffei* can differentiate into yeast cells and proliferate within alveolar macrophages [1]. The conversion of conidia to the yeast phase is the first critical process that permits *T. marneffei* to establish an infection, which is supported by the deletion of genes involved in phase transition altering the host response. The dimorphic transition of *T. marneffei* is a complex process involved by a number of genetic factors [31, 32].

According to the study of Yang *et al*. [33], the transcription factor *madsA* gene, a member of the MADS-box gene family, functions as a global regulator involved in the conidiation and germination, especially in the dimorphic transition of *T. marneffei*. In addition, overexpression of *madsA* in *T*. *marneffei* induced mycelium growth at 37°C, indicating that *madsA* is involved in the control of the dimorphic transition from yeast to mold. The deletion mutant and a complemented mutant of *madsA* in *T. marneffei* were then constructed and to identify its involvement in morphogenesis, dimorphic transition, and stress response [34]. When compared to the wild type and complementary strains, the Δ*madsA* demonstrated a faster transition from yeast (37°C) to mycelium (25°C) with abnormal morphogenesis. This study suggested that *madsA* functions as a regulator of yeast-to-mycelium transition and is closely related to conidiation and germination in *T. marneffei* although its roles in the survival, pathogenicity, and transmission require more investigation.

Despite the fact that temperature is only established stimulus controlling dimorphism in fungi, little study has been performed on the cellular changes or intracellular processes between the mycelial and yeast forms of *T. marneffei*. Based on yeast-phase specific proteins involved in virulence, the expression of yeast antigens of *T. marneffei* during phase transition was recently studied using a yeast-specific monoclonal antibody (MAb) 4D1 [35]. The MAb 4D1, yeast phase-specific MAb against *T. marneffei*, was produced using a modification of standard hybridoma technology with incorporating of cyclophosphamide without cross-reactivity to a panel of dimorphic and common fungal antigens [36, 37]. In addition, the MAb 4D1 was reactive against a 50–180 kDa broad high-molecular-weight smear of yeast phase mannoprotein antigen *in T. marneffei*. Recently, the MAb 4D1 was used to track cellular events in *T. marneffei* during phase transition and demonstrated that conidia were directly converted to fission yeast cells, with the expression of the yeast-specific antigen occurring 12 hours after phagocytosis by human THP-1 macrophage. These phenomena were clearly exhibited by overlapping signals between the green color of fluorescence isothiocyanate (FITC)-labeled conidia and the red color of MAb4D1 specific to yeast antigens, resulting in a yellow co-localized signal 12 hours after macrophage internalization

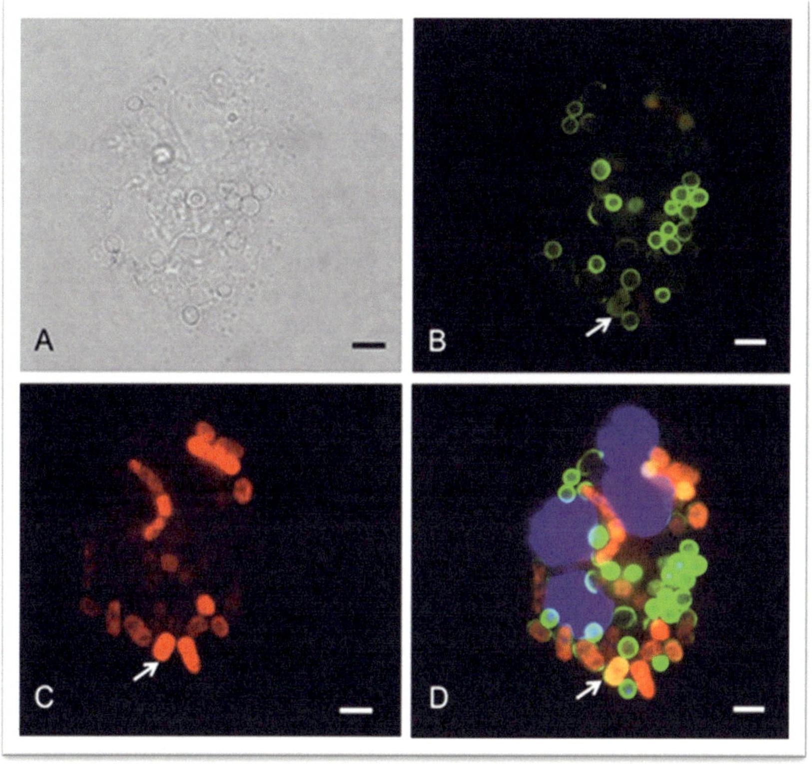

Figure 4.
The overlapping signals between the green of FITC-labeled conidia and the red of MAb4D1 which gives the co-localized signal as a yellow at 12 hours after internalization (white arrows). T. marneffei yeast cells were labeled with MAb 4D1 and Alexaflor 555-conjugated goat anti-mouse IgG antibody. A: Light microscopic image; B: Fluorescence image showing the green channel (FITC-labeled conidia); C: Fluorescence image of the red channel (MAb 4D1-positive yeast cells); D: THP-1 nuclei were stained with DAPI (blue) a merged channel showing the overlapping of images. Bars, 5 μm.

(**Figure 4**). When compared to the results in artificial cultivation media, this experiment demonstrated that the phase transitional ability of *T. marneffei* conidia in culture medium was converted to yeast cells at a slower rate than in the host macrophage THP-1 environment. Thus, MAb 4D1 can be applied as a biomolecular tool for understanding the phase transition of *T. marneffei* and provides strong evidence for this fungal shift from an environmental saprophyte to a pathogenic fungus.

The readily reversible nature of the mycelial to yeast and yeast to mycelial transformation processes in *T. marneffei* indicates that they are genetically controlled. A number of molecular biology studies have focused on the genetic factor that influences dimorphic switching in *T. marneffei*. Indeed, *abaA* expression is significantly upregulated during hyphal to yeast transformation in fungi [38]. The *abaA* deletion mutant also displays aberrant yeast morphology as both the developing transitory-state arthroconidial filaments and the yeast cells fail to couple nuclear and cellular division, resulting in multiple nuclei in both the arthroconidial compartments and yeast cells. Furthermore, during the yeast to mycelia transition, transient upregulation of expression of *cflA* [39] and *cflB* genes [40] was observed. However, mutations in these genes resulting in altered function to do not block the dimorphic property of *T. marneffei*. Further study has employed two-dimensional difference gel electrophoresis to investigate proteins expressed differently in the yeast and mycelial phases, as well as peptide mass fingerprinting to identify these *T. marneffei* differentially expressed proteins [41]. These two enzymes are required for *T. marneffei* to survive as yeast inside phagocytes, where it is protected from the host defense system. Isocitratelyase, in particular, is the key rate-limiting enzyme in the glyoxylate bypass, a metabolic pathway that supplements the tricarboxylic acid cycle and is required for the survival of some intracellular pathogenic fungi such as *P. brasiliensis* and *Cryptococcus neoformans* [42–44]. This demonstrates the requirement of *T. marneffei* in sustaining the glyoxylate cycle under the host's severe nutrient-depleted environment.

Transition to the yeast phase may provide protection from phagocyte destruction. Thermal dimorphism of this fungus plays an important role for survival in host phagocytes. However, the phenomenon that regulates this transit has remained an enigma. A number of molecular biology studies have concentrated upon the genetic element influenced in the dimorphic switching in *T. marneffei*. Many of those previously investigated including *stuA*, *stlA*, *gasA*, *gasC*, and *cflB* have no role in yeast cell development or the dimorphic switch. However, Borneman and his colleagues (2000) had found that *abaA* deletion mutant displayed aberrant mold to yeast conversion as both the developing transitory state arthroconidial filament and the yeast cells fail to couple nuclear and cell division, where multiple nuclei were observed within either arthroconidia or yeast cells. However, once conidia began to develop yeasts, a second series of genes appeared to take over the coupling of cell division events [38].

3.3 Oxidative stress response and heat-induced fungal adaptation proteins

Oxidative stress is one of the native defenses produced by the phagocytes to kill parasitic microorganisms. The phagocytes play a crucial role in eliminating fungal pathogens by producing reactive oxygen or nitrogen species, including superoxide radical anion (O^{2-}), hydrogen peroxide (H_2O_2), hydroxyl radicals (OH^-), and nitric oxide (NO) [45]. The reactive oxygen species (ROS) can damage pathogens by readily altering or inactivating proteins, membrane, nucleic acid, and they have potent immunoregulatory effects on the host immune system that affect the efficacy of the host response [46].

3.4 Catalase

Catalase peroxidase is capable of either reducing H_2O_2 with an external reductant or exchanging it to water and oxygen. The enzyme has been shown to be a virulence factor of *Mycobacterium tuberculosis* and *A. fumigatus* [47]. The catalase-peroxidase encoding gene (*CpeA*) in *T. marneffei* is associated with the upregulated expression of *CpeA* transcript both in yeast phase and under macrophage environment [48]. In recent years, Pongpom and her collaborators showed that *CpeA* controlled the fungus tolerance to H_2O_2 but not to heat stress response. H_2O_2 treatments induced high expression of this gene in both mold and yeast phase. It is therefore proposed that the *CpeA* of *T. marneffei* is utilized to protect the conidia and yeast cells from oxidative stress in the host macrophage environment [49].

3.5 Superoxide dismutase (SOD)

Superoxide dismutase (SOD) is an enzyme that alternately catalyzes the dismutation of the superoxide radical (O_2^-) into either ordinary molecular oxygen (O_2) or hydrogen peroxide (H_2O_2). *T. marneffei* has been shown to survive and replicate as yeast inside the macrophage phagosome. Previously, Thirach and her colleagues investigated the fungal superoxide dismutase encoding gene (*sodA*) and found that the putative SodA peptide consisted of 154 amino acid residues and shared identity to fungal copper, zinc superoxide dismutase. The results suggested that *sodA* might play a role in stress response and in the adaptation of *T. marneffei* inside the macrophage [50].

3.6 High-temperature-induced fungal adaptation proteins

Since the pathogenic phase of *T. marneffei* is closely linked with the higher temperature for normal growth in the environment, the heat-shock proteins (HSPs) are proposed as potential virulence factors. HSP always serve as a molecular chaperone, control protein folding, and transport intracellular proteins, as well as repair or destroy proteins. HSPs are a group of proteins produced by eukaryotic cells in response to exposure to stressful conditions, as they could be upregulated upon infection to prevent misfolding of damaged proteins [51]. The Hsp 70 of *T. marneffei* was first isolated and identified by Kummasook and colleagues (2007) [52]. The results showed that the *hsp70* transcription was upregulated during the mycelium to yeast transition. Upregulation was also observed when mycelial or yeast cells confronted to a heat stress environment at 39°C. It has been suggested that Hsp 70 may play an important role to prevent the yeast proteins from damage during temperature increase. Subsequently, Vanittanakom and her colleagues investigated the *hsp30* of this fungus and showed high transcription degree in yeast phase grown at 37°C, but undetectable transcript level was observed in mycelium phase at 25°C. These researchers suggested that Hsp 30 may play an important role in heat-shock response and in cellular adaptation during infection [53]. Based on the role of HSPs in temperature adaptation, the Hsp70 and Hsp 30 have definite functions in the host intracellular response; therefore, further study in *T. marneffei* is necessary.

3.7 Fungal melanin

Melanin is a high-molecular-weight dark brown or black pigment produced by oxidative polymerization of phenolic or indolic compounds. Melanins are produced by a wide range of organisms, including bacteria, fungi, plants, and animals. Although different types of melanins can be produced by fungal organisms, the majority of fungal melanins are 1,8-dihydroxynaph thalene (DHN) melanins and L-3,4-dihydroxyphenylalanine (DOPA) melanins [54]. In the DHN pathway, 1,3,6,8-tetrahydroxynaphthalene (1,3,6,8-THN), which is derived from acetyl-CoA or propionyl-CoA with malonyl-CoA or methylmalonyl-CoA, is the first product of a polyketide synthases (PKS) pathway. This compound is then sequentially converted to scytalone, 1,3,8-trihydroxynaphthalene (1,3,8-THN), vermelone, and lastly 1,8-DHN as demonstrated in **Figure 5** [55]. Finally, oxidative polymerization produces the end product, DHN-melanin [55]. The DHN melanin biosynthesis gene cluster of *T. marneffei* was studied [57]. A cluster of six-genes, *alb1*, *arp2*, *arp1*, *abr1*, *abr2*, and *ayg1* are associated with conidial pigment synthesis in this organism. The genes *alb1* (*pks4*), *arp1*, and *arp2* encode for a polyketide synthase (PKS), a scytalone dehydratase, and a 1,3,6,8-tetrahydroxynaphthalene reductase, while *abr1* and *abr2* appear to encode two oxidases, respectively. Furthermore, all of these genes are phylogenetically linked to the *A. fumigatus* counterparts, and the production of DHN-melanin in *T. marneffei* is thought to be comparable to that of *A. fumigatus* [58]. Tricyclazole

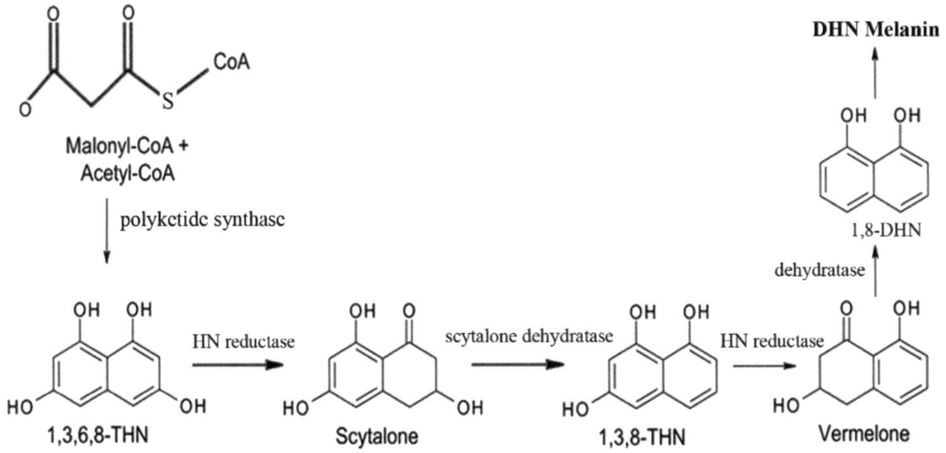

Figure 5.
Biosynthesis pathway of DHN melanin in fungi. Scheme adapted from [54–56].

which inhibits two hydroxynaphthalene reductases in the DHN-melanin synthesis pathway was used to confirm the DHN melanin of *T. marneffei* [59].

In *T. marneffei*, DOPA melanin is produced by yeast cells and composed of spherical granular particles in a beaded arrangement in the innermost cell wall [60, 61]. Bell and Wheeler [62] proposed a biosynthesis pathway for fungal DOPA melanin. There is experimental evidence for some of the proposed intermediates of that pathway [62–64]. In brief, laccase or tyrosinase catalyzes the hydroxylation of L-tyrosine to dopaquinone or the oxidation of L-DOPA to dopaquinone. Dopaquinone is a highly reactive intermediate which then forms leucodopachrome, which is oxidized to dopachrome. Hydroxylation (and decarboxylation) yields dihydroxyindoles that can polymerize to form DOPA melanin (**Figure 6**).

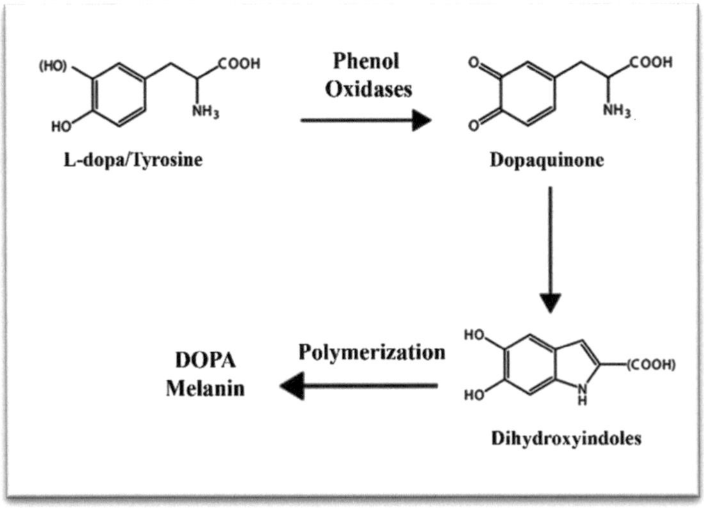

Figure 6.
The biosynthesis pathway of the dihydroxyphenylalanine (DOPA) melanin in fungi. Scheme adapted from [54, 56].

Both *T. marneffei* mycelial grown on culture medium at 25°C and yeast cells cultivated in a defined liquid minimal medium (MM) with L-DOPA were reactive with anti-melanin MAb 8D6, a melanin-binding MAb generated against *A. fumigatus* conidial melanin [60]. In mycelial phase, conidia, phialides, and hyphae were all positive with the anti-melanin MAb 8D6 (**Figure 7**). Thus, the melanization of *T. marneffei* was confirmed in both the mold and yeast forms.

Melanins have been influenced in virulence in many pathogenic fungi including *H. capsulatum*, *P. brasiliensis*, *C. neoformans*, *A. fumigatus* and *Sporothrix schenckii*. Melanin synthesis can help fungi survive in a variety of environments [65] and increase their resistance to host immune responses, such as reducing macrophage oxidative burst capacity [66], inhibiting apoptosis in macrophages [67], and inhibiting cytokine production in the host [68]. Youngchim and colleagues (2005) were the first to describe melanin in *T. marneffei*. The study demonstrated that melanins were produced both in *vitro* and during infection by presenting the melanization of yeast cells inside skin tissue from talaromycosis. Furthermore, sera from *T. marneffei* inoculated mice produced a significant antibody response against melanin, suggesting that melanin can act as an immunologically active molecule recognized by the immune

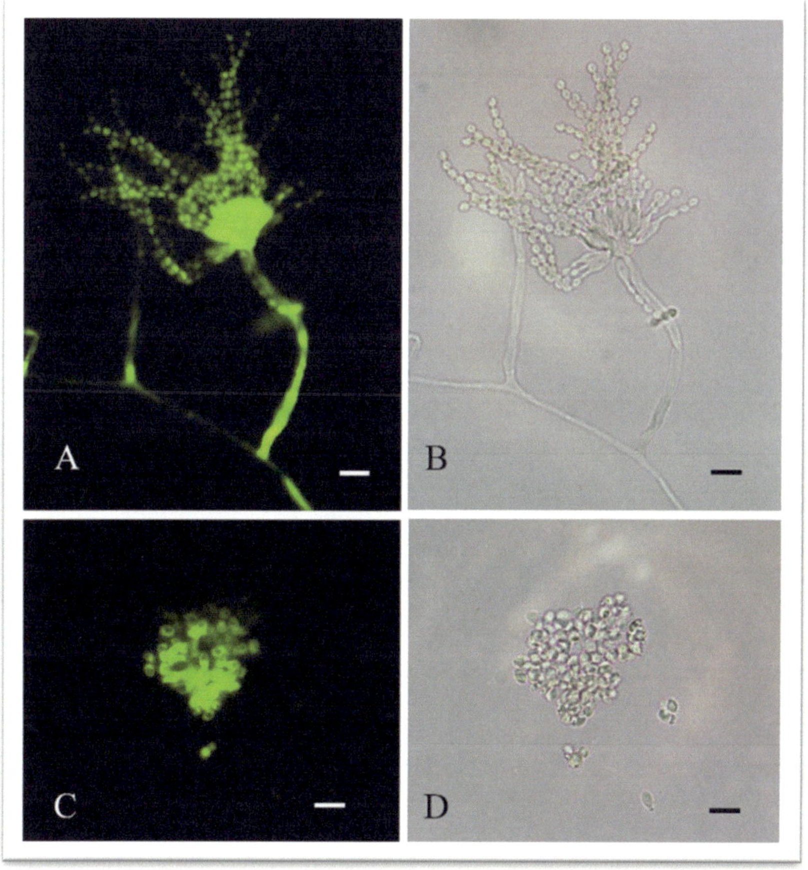

Figure 7.
The melanin production of T. marneffei *was detected in both mycelial and yeast forms using anti-melanin MAb 8D6. Corresponding immunofluorescence (A,C) and bright field (B,D) microscopy images demonstrating the labeling of mycelial phase (A,B) and yeast cells (C,D) of T. marneffei by anti-melanin MAb 8D6. Bar, 5 μm.*

system [69]. Melanin extracted from *T. marneffei* was also effective in inhibiting the production of TNF-α by the human monocyte cell line THP-1 indicating that melanin could conceal the organism from initial recognition by the immune system. In this respect, melanin is thought to contribute to *T. marneffei* virulence by allowing the organism to survive and grow within host tissue. The study of Woo *et al.* [70] confirmed that knocking down the melanin-biosynthesis gene cluster, *alb1*, in *T. marneffei* resulted in a loss of virulence in mice when compared to the wild type. The mutant also had a 50% reduction in conidial survival when exposed to hydrogen peroxide compared to the wild type. In fact, melanin has been named "an antifungal resistance factor" due to its ability to make melanized cells less susceptible to antifungal drugs [71, 72]. It was confirmed from our previous study that melanin appears to protect *T. marneffei* by making it more resistant to antifungal drugs including amphotericin B, clotrimazole, fluconazole, itraconazole, and ketoconazole [73].

The melanin produced by *T. marneffei* may play some roles in the virulence factor of this fungus. Melanin acts as a power protector for *T. marneffei in vitro* by decreasing phagocytosis and increasing resistance to macrophage intracellular digestion [61]. Interestingly, heat-shock proteins (HSPs), particularly HSP90 in *T. Marneffei*, were found to be significantly more expressed in DOPA melanin yeast cells compared to non-melanized yeast cells using proteomic analysis [74]. By making further analysis in the proteomic pathway, heat-shock proteins were enriched in multiple important metabolic pathways, including stress response pathway and phagosome development indicating that HSP90 plays an important role in melanin synthesis pathway of *T. marneffei*.

3.8 Fungal laccase

P-diphenol dioxygen oxidoreductases or laccases are multi-copper containing oxidoreductase that catalyzed the oxidation of organic and inorganic substances including phenol containing amino acid, methoxy phenol, and aromatics amine, with the concomitant 4 electrons reduction of oxygen to water [75]. The essential properties of fungal laccases have been investigated and were shown to influence fungal development, to control phenotype and morphogenesis, to detoxify toxins, and to control pathogenesis in pathogenic fungi and stress response adaptation [76]. Laccases have been associated as contributors to virulence in many fungal pathogens such as *A. fumigatus* and *C. neoformans.* In *C. neoformans*, this enzyme can also promote the pathogenicity of *C. neoformans* by catalyzing the formation of melanin precursors. Melanized *C. neoformans* cell were more negatively charged on the cell wall, and this phenomenon could interfere with the phagocytosis mechanism [71]. The role of laccases in the virulence factor and pathogenesis in *T. marneffei* were characterized by Sapmak and colleagues [77]. It was found that quadruple deletions of laccase encoding genes (*lac1, lac2, lac3*, and *arb2*) in *T. marneffei* mutant were more sensitive to oxidative stressor, cell wall stressor, and antifungal agents including itraconazole, fluconazole, and clotrimazole. Subsequently, the results showed that the mutant strain of *T. marneffei* was more susceptible to killing by human macrophages, THP-1, than the wild-type *T. marneffei*. Moreover, the observation on the pro-inflammatory cytokine production in THP-1 human macrophages showed that the mutant *T. marneffei* stimulated a significantly higher production of TNF-α, IL-1β, and IL-6 compared to the wild type. Altogether, these results defined the role of laccases that influenced *T. marneffei* resistance to the host immune response [77].

3.9 Fungal cell wall, mannoproteins Mp1p

The fungal cell wall is a critical structure with high flexibility that is important for cellular integrity and vitality. Mannoproteins are one of the most important structural components of the fungal cell wall. In fact, substantial study with yeast has demonstrated that mannoproteins perform a variety of biological functions, including defining cell shape, stimulating cell growth and morphological change, functioning as a protective factor, aiding sex agglutination, and regulating cell wall porosity [78–81]. Mp1p is an antigenic cell wall mannoprotein found in yeast, hyphae, and conidia of *T. marneffei* and has been effectively employed in serodiagnosis and infection prevention [57, 82–85]. Mp1p is a 462-amino-acid protein having three domains: ligand-binding domain 1 (LBD1), ligand-binding domain 2 (LBD2), and a serine and threonine-rich domain near the C terminus [84]. Mp1p is a new virulence factor of *T. marneffei* through knockout and knockdown research employing an intracellular survival assay with murine macrophage cells and mice challenge models [86]. For a mouse model, the mice could live for up to 60 days without talaromycosis after being challenged with a Mp-knockout strain of *T. marneffei*, but the wild-type strain killed the mice within 21 days. In addition, the organ fungal burden and inflammatory response in mice infected with the MP1 knockout mutant were significantly reduced compared to the wild type.

Based on the structure of Mp1p, Mp1p-LBD2, a ligand-binding domain, is a strong arachidonic acid (AA) binder by forming a five-helix bundle monomeric structure with a long hydrophobic central cavity for high-affinity encapsulation of cellular AA [87]. AA is a key pro-inflammatory mediator because it is produced as a main eicosanoid precursor in response to microbial infection, which can generate many downstream prostaglandins and common markers of pro-inflammatory responses, including TNF-α and IL-6 [88]. Subsequently, Lam *et al.* [89] demonstrated that not only Mp1p-LBD2, but Mp1p-LBD1 is also a strong AA-binding domain in Mp1p. Thus, Mp1p is an effective AA-capturing protein that uses two AA-binding domains, Mp1p-LBD1 and Mp1p-LBD2, to capture released AA during the early stages of pro-inflammatory reactions. According to the crystal structure, Mp1p-LBD1-LBD2 are likely to function independently and equally important in terms of AA capturing, with each domain capable of accommodating two AA molecules. Taken together, Mp1p represents a novel class of fatty acid-binding proteins with the function of targeting key pro-inflammatory signaling lipid to suppress the host innate immune response.

3.10 Iron and calcium are essential cations required for growth and virulence

Ca^{2+} signaling plays an essential role in various processes, including cation homeostasis, pH adaptation, glucose metabolism, morphogenesis, and virulence in fungi [30, 90]. The Ca^{2+}-binding protein calmodulin and the Ca^{2+}/calmodulin-dependent phosphatase calcineurin are two major mediators of calcium signals in eukaryotic cells [91]. Calcineurin is a serine/threonine phosphatase that composed of two subunits of catalytic (CnaA) and regulatory (CnaB) that is activated through the binding of Ca^{2+}-calmodulin (CaM) [92].

Calcineurin plays a crucial role in fungal virulence such as *A. fumigatus* [93, 94], *C. neoformans* [95], *Candida* spp. [96–98] and *Pacoccidiodes brasiliensis* [99]. Recent studies reveal a role of calcineurin in growth and virulence of *T. marneffei* [100]. In *T. marneffei*, deletion of the *cnaA* gene resulted in substantial defects in conidiation, germination, morphogenesis, cell wall integrity, and tolerance to several stresses.

The importance of calcineurin functions in cell wall integrity of *T. marneffei* was supported by the study of MICs against caspofungin and micafungin, which revealed lower MICs in the *cnaA* mutant when compared to wild type. These two antifungal agents belong to the echinocandins that inhibit fungal cell wall biosynthesis by inhibiting cell wall β-(1,3)-D glucan synthesis [101]. In addition, the *cnaA* mutant conidia were not only more susceptible to salt, H_2O_2, and osmotic stress *in vitro*, but they also rarely germinated or processed yeast morphogenesis after being phagocytosed by macrophages. Calcineurin is also required for full virulence in a murine model of invasive *T. marneffei* infection. Thus, calcineurin homolog (*cnaA*) regulates fungal morphogenesis and the response of *T. marneffei* to external stressors, as well as the host immunological response and fungal pathogenicity.

Iron is an important trace element that is often limited for pathogens during infection; hence, adaptability to iron deficiency is critical for virulence [102, 103]. Indeed, iron has been demonstrated to be essential for *T. marneffei* development and pathogenicity. Iron overload also significantly decreased the antifungal activity of macrophages [104]. As *T. marneffei* lacks an iron excretion mechanism, controlling iron uptake, metabolism, and regulation can play an important role in iron homeostasis. Fungi have developed two methods to get iron in iron-limited environments: reductive iron assimilation (RIA) and siderophore-mediated iron acquisition [105, 106]. RIA begins with the reduction of ferric iron sources to more soluble ferrous iron by plasma membrane-localized ferrireductases [107]. Then, the ferrous iron is re-oxidized and imported by a protein complex composed of the ferroxidase, FetC, and the iron permease, FtrA. Both *fetC* and *ftrA* gene expression was higher in yeast cells (37°C) than in hyphal cells (25°C) with a clear upregulation in response to iron limitation [108]. Deletion of *ftrA* results in a defective RIA system, which reduces the growth of yeast cells but not hyphal cells under low iron conditions [109]. For siderophore biosynthesis pathway, *sidD* and *sidF* genes involved in the biosynthesis of extracellular siderophores of *T. marneffei* were upregulated early during yeast morphogenesis switching from 25 to 37°C and late during yeast cell growth [108].

Based on the functions of *sidA* and *sidX*, these two genes encoded the enzyme ornithine N5-oxygenase, which catalyzed ornithine to hydroxyornithine in an early step of the siderophore biosynthesis pathway. SidA is involved in extracellular siderophore formation in the mycelial phase, whereas SidX is involved in both intracellular and extracellular siderophore production in the yeast phase [109]. Mutant analysis revealed that *T. marneffei* yeast cells can utilize RIA for iron acquisition, providing another system in this cell type that varies extensively from hyphal cells. For example, the expression of *fetC* (involved in RIA) was significantly elevated in Δ*sidA* and Δ*sidX* yeast cells but not in hyphal cells.

Furthermore, *T. marneffei* has recently been studied for the expression of *acuM* and *acuK*, which have been found to be involved in gluconeogenesis and iron metabolism [110]. In fact, *AcuM* and *AcuK* are homologous Zn2Cys6 transcription factors previously identified as gluconeogenesis and iron metabolism regulators in other pathogenic fungi such as *A. nidulans* [111] and *A. fumigatus* [112]. *T. marneffei* transcript levels of *acuM* and *acuK* were sequentially downregulated when the fungus was grown in increasing iron concentrations [110]. As a result, the transcription factors AcuM and AcuK may play a role in iron metabolism by either reducing iron uptake or alleviating iron toxicity. In contrast, the *acuM* transcript was upregulated in the gluconeogenic condition, but the *acuK* transcript was only elevated in the acetate medium during the yeast phase. Taken together, the genes *acuM* and *acuK* have been linked to iron homeostasis and gluconeogenesis in *T. marneffei*. Deletion of *acuK* gene in *T. marneffei* resulted in a growth defect under iron-deficient conditions since the mutant produced fewer siderophores [113]. The *fetC* transcript in ΔacuK was significantly increased than in the wild type, indicating that *acuK* may be a negative regulator of *fetC* expression, the gene encoding an RIA enzyme in *T. marneffei*. In contrast, the *sidA* and *sidX* transcripts involved in the first step of siderophore biosynthesis in Δ*acuK* were relatively low. This finding implied that *sidA* and *sidX* may be controlled by Acuk, and the detailed mechanism has yet to be investigated. As iron assimilation is the complex system, more studies are required to completely understand its regulation mechanism.

3.11 Extracellular vesicles (EVs)

Extracellular vesicles (EVs), a type of nanoscale lipid bilayer membrane structure, play a function in transporting molecules to the extracellular space and are referred to as "virulence bags" [114, 115]. The characteristics and potential roles of these vesicles in virulence have been studied in a number of pathogenic fungi such as *C. neoformans*, *C. albicans*, *H. capsulatum*, and *P. brasiliensis* [116–119].

In *T. marneffei*, EVs had a typical spherical shape with a diameter of 30 to 300 nm under the nanoparticle tracking analysis (NTA) and TEM [120]. The functions of EVs released by *T. marneffei* could promote the expression levels of reactive oxygen species (ROS), nitric oxide, and some inflammatory factors including interleukin-1β, interleukin-6, interleukin-10, and tumor necrosis factor in RAW 264.7 macrophage cells. It was also reported that *T. marneffei* could secrete EVs loaded with some active molecules including heat-shock protein, mannoprotein 1 (MP1p), and peroxidase. As an important carrier containing a variety of molecules, EVs play a crucial role in intercellular communication with host immune responses.

4. Laboratory diagnosis of talaromycosis

4.1 Staining and culture methods

Microbiological culture and histological staining are commonly used for diagnosis of *T. marneffei* infection. Clinical specimens including bone marrows aspirates, lymph node biopsies, blood, sputum, pleural fluid, cerebrospinal fluid (CSF), urine, and liver biopsies were used for diagnosis of *T. marneffei* infection [11, 121]. In addition, Wright's staining of bone marrows aspirates and touch smear of skin biopsy or lymph node biopsies is a rapid diagnostic method [122] (**Figure 8**). The fungus can be seen in histological sections stained with Grocott methenamine silver (GMS) or periodic acid–Schiff (PAS). In contrast, *T. marneffei* yeast cells may result in the false impression that a capsule mimics to *H. capsulatum* when staining with hematoxylin and eosin (H&E) [123].

Microbiological cultivation is a gold standard for diagnosis of talaromycosis. The bone marrows gave the highest yield for culture positive, approaching 100%, followed by culture of other specimens obtained from skin biopsy (90%) and hemoculture (76%) [11]. However, most of the fungal isolates in microbiological laboratory screening are usually obtained from hemoculture of HIV-infected patients and need to confirm the dimorphic transition of this fungus. *T. marneffei* was confirmed by morphology and thermal dimorphism. *T. marneffei* was confirmed by macroscopic and microscopic examination. However, a limitation of the culture method is time-consuming, taking about 1 to 2 weeks. Given that ineffective

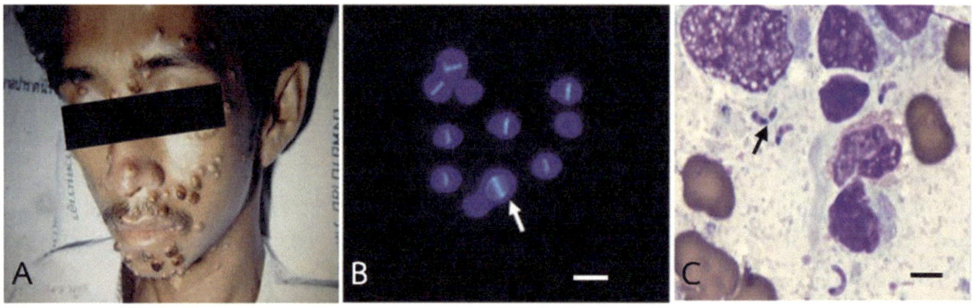

Figure 8.
Typical disfiguring central-umbilicated skin lesions on the face of a patient with advanced HIV and disseminated talaromycosis in Thailand (A), calcofluor white stained touch skin smear, showing fission yeast cells (B) and sausage-shaped yeasts with binary fission outside macrophage (C). The arrow heads highlight the midline septum in a dividing yeast cell characteristic of T. marneffei. Scale bar represents 5 μm.

fungal therapy of *T. marneffei* is associated with poor prognosis and can be fatal, more rapid diagnosis of infection is preferable.

4.2 Serodiagnosis

Many serodiagnostic assays have been developed for the detection of *T. marneffei* antigen from various clinical specimens, as shown in **Table 2**. Based on a potent immunogenic protein known as Mp1p, the protein is made up of galactomannoprotein which located throughout the cell wall of *T. marneffei* yeast [85, 123] have developed monoclonal antibodies (MAbs) and polyclonal antibodies (PAbs) against cell wall mannoprotein Mp1p expressed in *Pichia pastoris*. These antibodies were applied to detect antigens by using antigen capture ELISA. The method exhibited the sensitivities and specificities of 55% and 99.6% for the MAbs-MAbs based method and 75% and 99.4% for the MAbs-PAbs based method. There was no cross-reactivity found in 11 common pathogenic fungi, including *Cryptococcus*, *Candida*, *Aspergillus*, and *Histoplasma*. The Mp1p EIA was then applied to plasma samples of 372 patients who had culture-proven talaromycosis from blood and 517 individuals without talaromycosis (338 healthy volunteers and 179 with other infections) in Vietnam, demonstrating 98.1% specificity and 86.3% sensitivity [124]. In addition, paired plasma and urine testing in the same patients (n = 269) significantly improved sensitivity when compared to testing plasma or urine alone.

The most recent antigen detection assays developed for the diagnosis of *T. marneffei* infection have demonstrated the potential diagnostic application of MAb 4D1 [36]. In addition, MAb 4D1 (an IgG1) recognizes a 50–180 kDa manoproteins and the MAb shows specificity without cross-reactivity to a panel of dimorphic and common fungal antigens. Then, a new inhibitory ELISA using MAb 4D1 was designed to determine the antigenic concentration of *T. marneffei* in patient sera. The test identified antigenemia in all 45 (100%) talaromycosis, with a mean antigen concentration of 4.32 μg/ml. No cross-reactivity in this assay was found in patients with other fungal or bacterial infections, and healthy controls. This result showed that the detection of circulating antigens in talaromycosis was beneficially useful not only for diagnostic purposes but also as a tool to evaluate the clearance of fungal burden during treatment.

Currently, there is no commercially available diagnostic kit for talaromycosis. The available alternative serodiagnostic method for talaromycosis in routine laboratory

#	Methods	Diagnostic antigen	Diagnostic sensitivity*	Diagnostic specificity**
1	Immunodiffusion (microimmuno-diffusion)	Exoantigen	25 (2/8)	N/A
2	Immunodiffusion	Fission arthroconidia filtrate	11.7% (2/17)	100% (0/40)
3	Indirect immunofluorescent assay	Germinating conidia and yeast—hyphae cells	100%(8/8) IgG titer >160	N/A
4	Immunoblotting	Secreted yeast early stationary phase exoantigen profiles	200 kDa: 72.7% (24/33) 88 kDa: 94% (31/33) 54 kDa: 60.6% (20/33) 50 kDa: 57.6% (19/33)	200 kDa: 79.3% (23/29) 88 kDa: 93.1% (27/29) 54 kDa: 13.8% (4/29) 50 kDa: 10.8% (3/29) (for AIDS patients without Talaromycosis)
5	Immunoblotting	38 kDa of mycelial cell culture filtrate	45% (23/51)	28% (11/39) cross- reacted with Cryptococcosis 21% (6/28) cross- reacted with Candidiasis
6	Immunoblotting	Cytoplasmic yeast antigen (TM CYA) profiles	61 kDa: 48% (10/21) 54 kDa: 71% (15/21) 50 kDa: 48% (10/21) 86% (18/21) Recognized at least one bandof TM CYA	100% (0/80)
7	Indirect ELISA	Recombinant fusion Mp1p (expressed in *Escherichia coli)*	82% (14/17)	100% (0/165)
8	Immunoblotting	Recombinant Mplp6	95% (19/20)	100% (0/35)
9	Immunoblotting	Recombinant Hsp30 fusion protein	20% (2/10)	100% (0/10)
10	Indirect Mp1p IgG ELISA	Recombinant Mp1p (expressed in *Pichia pastoris*)	30% (6/20)	98.5% (532/540)

Footnote

N/A: No data or inconclusive data
**Compared with culture confirmed talaromycosis*
***Compared with other microorganism infection, healthy individual living in endemic area and asymptomatic HIV infection living in endemic area*

Table 2.
Summarized immunological methods for detection of T. marneffei specific antibodies.

is based on Platelia *Aspergillus* EIA which is designed for the detection of circulating *A. fumigatus* GM antigens. It has been reported that the GM antigens of *T. marneffei and Aspergillus* are very similar, and the EIA test could therefore give high degree of diagnostic sensitivity for talaromycosis [20, 125]. As a result, the intimate concordance rate between Mp1p antigen detection and the GM antigen assay in antigenemia of talaromycosis was demonstrated, which is extremely important. Several studies have revealed significant false-positive due to the cross-reaction of the MAb against GM (Rat MAb EB-A2) with GM antigen from non-*Aspergillus* spp., e.g. *Geotrichum capitatum*, *H. capsulatum*, *P. brasiliensis*, *B. dermatitidis*, *Mycobacterium tuberculosis*, galactoxylomannan from *C. neoformans*, and *C. gattii* and serum of patient treated with piperacillin-tazobactam or amoxicillin-clavulanic acid. It is not surprising that GM antigen is a "Pan-specific" marker for the fungal infection. Similarity between the (1–3)-β-D-glucan (BG) or "Fungitell" has been used for the diagnosis of filamentous fungal infections [126]. However, the lack of specificity means was unable to discriminate between *Aspergillus* spp. and other pathogenic fungi.

4.3 Rapid lateral flow immunochromatographic assay (ICA)

Recently, the rapid lateral flow ICAs have been developed for immunodiagnosis of the infection due to the clinically important fungi, e.g. polysaccharide antigen detection for *C. neoformans* [127], detection of specific IgG against *Pythium insidiosum* [128], hyphal-specific antigen detection of *Candida* species [129], and MAb against secreted glycoprotein of *A. fumigatus* for the diagnosis of invasive aspergillosis [130].

A "point-of-care" diagnosis of talaromycosis is urgently needed [2, 131]. Recently, we demonstrated a novel inhibition format of an ICT strip for rapid detection of the *T. marneffei* antigen from clinical urine samples. In this study, *T. marneffei* cytoplasmic yeast antigens (TM CYA) and the corresponding MAb 4D1 conjugated with nanoparticles of gold colloid were used. The inhibition (inh)-ICT strip was evaluated for its diagnostic performance in urine samples from both talaromycosis patients and a control group. The inh-ICT was highly specific against antigenuria from *T. marneffei* only, and it did not detect antigenuria of other clinically important microorganisms. The limit of the detection was 3.12 μg/mL of fungal antigen. The inh-ICT was used to test urine samples from 66 patients with confirmed *T. marneffei* infection, 40 patients with other microbial infections, and 72 healthy individuals from endemic area. The test exhibited diagnostic sensitivity, specificity, and accuracy of 87.87%, 100%, and 95.50%, respectively, for *T. marneffei* [132]. However, the Inh-ICT has some limitations on the relatively low diagnostic sensitivity and occasional ambiguity in the reading and interpretation of the observed results. The innovative sandwich ICT strip was created to improve the diagnostic efficiency of ICT strips by using a mannose binding lectin, which recognizes mannose residue called *Galanthus nivalis* agglutinin (GNA) or snowdrop lectin, in conjunction with MAb 4D1 [133]. The MAb4D1-GNA-based ICT showed specific binding activity with yeast phase antigen of *T. marneffei*, and it did not react with other common pathogenic fungal antigens. The diagnostic performance of the ICT was validated using 341 urine samples from patents with culture-confirmed *T. marneffei* infection and from a control group of healthy individuals and patients with other infections in an endemic area resulting 89.47% sensitivity, 100% specificity, and 97.65% accuracy. As a result, the *T. marneffei* ICT should be evaluated for clinical use in the context of rapid and affordable point-of-care diagnostic test to reduce the burden of talaromycosis mortality in patients in low-income countries.

4.4 Molecular diagnosis

The polymerase chain reaction (PCR) has been utilized effectively for the specific detection of many pathogenic fungi. The nucleotide primer PM2 and PM4 have been developed to amplify a 347 bp fragment of the internal transcribed spacer (ITS) element between 18 s rRNA and 5.8 s rRNA [134]. Novel oligonucleotide probes RRF1 and RRH1 were used in PCR southern hybridization format for the amplification of a 631 bp. fragment of the 18 s rRNA and then hybridized with a *T. marneffei* specific 15 oligonucleotide probes [135]. Further molecular diagnosis method was described; a one tube seminested PCR assay based on the 18 s rRNA region was developed to identify *T. marneffei* genome [136]. This method was useful and can detect *T. marneffei* DNA both from culture and clinical samples. An additional nested PCR test and a real-time PCR assay were used to detect *T. marneffei* in whole blood samples. Given the high sensitivity of nested PCR (82%) and real-time PCR (91%), the combination of these two PCR methods provides an interesting alternative for identifying *T. marneffei* DNA in whole blood samples [137]. However, these methods need the clinician establishing a hypothesis before to examination. *T. marneffei* is an uncommon pathogen in non-HIV individuals, particularly in areas outside of Southeast Asia where detection and therapy of talaromycosis may be restricted. Next-generation sequencing (NGS) based on metagenomics has recently been used to successfully diagnose disseminated *T. marneffei* infection. Under these conditions, the use of mNGS enabled for the rapid and accurate diagnosis of *T. marneffei* without the requirement for specified problematic pathogens, which is a proven advantage in talaromycosis diagnosis, resulting in improved individual patient treatment [138, 139]. At the time, the cost is the major hindrance to its wide usage. If the cost of NGS is reduced further and expertise is made more widely available, it will be an effective instrument in the repertoire for laboratory diagnosis of *T. marneffei* infection.

5. Conclusion

Talaromyces (previously *Penicillium*) marneffei causes a life-threatening invasive mycosis both in immunocompromised and immunocompetent individuals living in tropical and subtropical Asia. *T. marneffei* can adapt and express many virulence factors to survive inside hosts and then infect in those patients. The current understanding of the dynamic interaction between *T. marneffei* and its mammalian hosts emphasizes the role of virulence factors, such as adhesion to host tissue, dimorphic switching, oxidative responses, heat-shock protein, and melanin, which allowed the pathogen to evade host immune cells. Diagnosis of talaromycosis is frequently delayed which can result in unnecessary antibiotic use, unnecessary hospital admissions, and increased morbidity and mortality. Conventional methods of diagnosis have relied on the culture or examination of fungi; however, the time required to obtain results from culture and the lack of sensitivity of visual inspection tests can make them inconvenient. Thus, rapid diagnosis frequently based on antigen testing can help with the identification of talaromycosis.

Conflict of interest

The author declares no conflict of interest.

Author details

Sirida Youngchim
Department of Microbiology, Faculty of Medicine, Chiang Mai University,
Chiang Mai, Thailand

*Address all correspondence to: syoungchim@gmail.com

References

[1] Vanittanakom N, Cooper CR Jr, Fisher MC, Sirisanthana T. *Penicillium marneffei* infection and recent advances in the epidemiology and molecular biology aspects. Clinical Microbiology Reviews. 2006;**19**(1):95-110

[2] Limper AH, Adenis A, Le T, Harrison TS. Fungal infections in HIV/AIDS. The Lancet Infectious Diseases. 2017;**17**(11):e334-e343

[3] Hu Y, Zhang J, Li X, Yang Y, Zhang Y, Ma J, et al. *Penicillium marneffei* infection: An emerging disease in mainland China. Mycopathologia. 2013;**175**(1-2):57-67

[4] Antinori S, Gianelli E, Bonaccorso C, Ridolfo AL, Croce F, Sollima S, et al. Disseminated *Penicillium marneffei* infection in an HIV-positive Italian patient and a review of cases reported outside endemic regions. Journal of Travel Medicine. 2006;**13**(3):181-188

[5] Castro-Lainez MT, Sierra-Hoffman M, et al. *Talaromyces marneffei* infection in a non-HIV non-endemic population. IDCases. 2018;**12**:21-24

[6] Julander I, Petrini B. *Penicillium marneffei* infection in a Swedish HIV-infected immunodeficient narcotic addict. Scandinavian Journal of Infectious Diseases. 1997;**29**(3):320-322

[7] De Monte A, Risso K, Normand AC, Boyer G, L'Ollivier C, Marty P, et al. Chronic pulmonary penicilliosis due to *Penicillium marneffei*: Late presentation in a french traveler. Journal of Travel Medicine. 2014;**21**(4):292-294

[8] Patassi AA, Saka B, Landoh DE, Kotosso A, Mawu K, Halatoko WA, et al. First observation in a non-endemic country (Togo) of *Penicillium marneffei* infection in a human immunodeficiency virus-infected patient: A case report. BMC Research Notes. 2013;**6**:506

[9] Pautler KB, Padhye AA, Ajello L. Imported penicilliosis marneffei in the United States: Report of a second human infection. Sabouraudia. 1984;**22**(5):433-438

[10] Li L, Chen K, Dhungana N, Jang Y, Chaturvedi V, Desmond E. Characterization of clinical isolates of *Talaromyces marneffei* and related species, California, USA. Emerging Infectious Diseases. 2019;**25**(9):1765-1768

[11] Supparatpinyo K, Khamwan C, Baosoung V, Nelson KE, Sirisanthana T. Disseminated *Penicillium marneffei* infection in Southeast Asia. Lancet. 1994;**344**(8915):110-113

[12] Chariyalertsak S, Sirisanthana T, Saengwonloey O, Nelson KE. Clinical presentation and risk behaviors of patients with acquired immunodeficiency syndrome in Thailand, 1994-1998: Regional variation and temporal trends. Clinical Infectious Diseases. 2001;**32**(6):955-962

[13] Sun HY, Chen MY, Hsiao CF, Hsieh SM, Hung CC, Chang SC. Endemic fungal infections caused by *Cryptococcus neoformans* and *Penicillium marneffei* in patients infected with human immunodeficiency virus and treated with highly active anti-retroviral therapy. Clinical Microbiology and Infection. 2006;**12**(4):381-388

[14] Chan JF, Lau SK, Yuen KY, Woo PC. *Talaromyces (Penicillium) marneffei* infection in non-HIV-infected patients. Emerging Microbes Infection. 2016;**5**:e19

[15] Le T, Farrar J, Shikuma C. Rebound of plasma viremia following cessation of antiretroviral therapy despite profoundly low levels of HIV reservoir: Implications for eradication. AIDS. 2011;**25**(6):871-872

[16] Shen Q, Sheng L, Zhang J, Ye J, Zhou J. Analysis of clinical characteristics and prognosis of talaromycosis (with or without human immunodeficiency virus) from a non-endemic area: A retrospective study. Infection. 2022;**50**(1):169-178

[17] Kawila R, Chaiwarith R, Supparatpinyo K. Clinical and laboratory characteristics of penicilliosis marneffei among patients with and without HIV infection in Northern Thailand: A retrospective study. BMC Infectious Diseases. 2013;**13**:464

[18] Cao C, Xi L, Chaturvedi V. Talaromycosis (Penicilliosis) due to *Talaromyces (Penicillium) marneffei*: Insights into the clinical trends of a major fungal disease 60 years after the discovery of the pathogen. Mycopathologia. 2019;**184**(6):709-720

[19] Ajello L, Padhye AA, Sukroongreung S, Nilakul CH, Tantimavanic S. Occurrence of *Penicillium marneffei* infections among wild bamboo rats in Thailand. Mycopathologia. 1995;**131**(1):1-8

[20] Huang X, He G, Lu S, Liang Y, Xi L. Role of *Rhizomys pruinosus* as a natural animal host of *Penicillium marneffei* in Guangdong, China. Microbes Biotechnology. 2015;**8**(4):659-664

[21] Chariyalertsak S, Sirisanthana T, Supparatpinyo K, Nelson KE. Seasonal variation of disseminated *Penicillium marneffei* infections in northern Thailand: A clue to the reservoir? The Journal of Infectious Diseases. 1996;**173**(6):1490-1493

[22] Vossler J. *Penicillium marneffei*: An emerging fungal pathogen. Clinical Microbiology. 2001;**23**:25-29

[23] Coulot P, Bouchara JP, Renier G, Annaix V, Planchenault C, Tronchin G, et al. Specific interaction of *Aspergillus fumigatus* with fibrinogen and its role in cell adhesion. Infection and Immunity. 1994;**62**(6):2169-2177

[24] Gil ML, Penalver MC, Lopez-Ribot JL, O'Connor JE, Martinez JP. Binding of extracellular matrix proteins to *Aspergillus fumigatus* conidia. Infection and Immunity. 1996;**64**(12):5239-5247

[25] Mittal J, Ponce MG, Gendlina I, Nosanchuk JD. *Histoplasma capsulatum*: Mechanisms for pathogenesis. Current Topics in Microbiology and Immunology. 2019;**422**:157-191

[26] Hamilton AJ, Jeavons L, Youngchim S, Vanittanakom N. Recognition of fibronectin by *Penicillium marneffei* conidia via a sialic acid-dependent process and its relationship to the interaction between conidia and laminin. Infection and Immunity. 1999;**67**(10):5200-5205

[27] Hamilton AJ, Jeavons L, Youngchim S, Vanittanakom N, Hay RJ. Sialic acid-dependent recognition of laminin by *Penicillium marneffei* conidia. Infection and Immunity. 1998;**66**(12):6024-6026

[28] Srinoulprasert Y, Kongtawelert P, Chaiyaroj SC. Chondroitin sulfate B and heparin mediate adhesion of *Penicillium marneffei* conidia to host extracellular matrices. Microbial Pathogenesis. 2006;**40**(3):126-132

[29] Lau SK, Tse H, Chan JS, Zhou AC, Curreem SO, Lau CC, et al. Proteome profiling of the dimorphic fungus *Penicillium marneffei* extracellular proteins and identification of

glyceraldehyde-3-phosphate dehydrogenase as an important adhesion factor for conidial attachment. The FEBS Journal. 2013;**280**(24):6613-6626

[30] Boyce KJ, Andrianopoulos A. Fungal dimorphism: The switch from hyphae to yeast is a specialized morphogenetic adaptation allowing colonization of a host. FEMS Microbiology Reviews. 2015;**39**(6):797-811

[31] Andrianopoulos A. Control of morphogenesis in the human fungal pathogen *Penicillium marneffei*. International Journal of Medical Microbiology. 2002;**292**(5-6):331-347

[32] Boyce KJ, Andrianopoulos A. Morphogenetic circuitry regulating growth and development in the dimorphic pathogen *Penicillium marneffei*. Eukaryotic Cell. 2013;**12**(2):154-160

[33] Yang E, Chow WN, Wang G, Woo PC, Lau SK, Yuen KY, et al. Signature gene expression reveals novel clues to the molecular mechanisms of dimorphic transition in *Penicillium marneffei*. PLoS Genetics. 2014;**10**(10):e1004662

[34] Wang Q, Du M, Wang S, Liu L, Xiao L, Wang L, et al. MADS-Box transcription factor *MadsA* regulates dimorphic transition, conidiation, and germination of *Talaromyces marneffei*. Frontiers in Microbiology. 2018;**9**:1781

[35] Pruksaphon K, Intaramat A, Ratanabanangkoon K, Nosanchuk JD, Vanittanakom N, Youngchim S. Diagnostic laboratory immunology for talaromycosis (penicilliosis): Review from the bench-top techniques to the point-of-care testing. Diagnostic Microbiology and Infectious Disease. 2020;**96**(3):114959

[36] Prakit K, Nosanchuk JD, Pruksaphon K, Vanittanakom N, Youngchim S. A novel inhibition ELISA for the detection and monitoring of *Penicillium marneffei* antigen in human serum. European Journal of Clinical Microbiology & Infectious Diseases. 2016;**35**(4):647-656

[37] Rafferty K. *Penicillium marneffei*: Immunological Response to Infection and Development of Novel Diagnostic Methods. London, UK: University of London; 2004

[38] Borneman AR, Hynes MJ, Andrianopoulos A. The *abaA* homologue of *Penicillium marneffei* participates in two developmental programmes: Conidiation and dimorphic growth. Molecular Microbiology. 2000;**38**(5):1034-1047

[39] Boyce KJ, Hynes MJ, Andrianopoulos A. The CDC42 homolog of the dimorphic fungus *Penicillium marneffei* is required for correct cell polarization during growth but not development. Journal of Bacteriology. 2001;**183**(11):3447-3457

[40] Boyce KJ, Hynes MJ, Andrianopoulos A. Control of morphogenesis and actin localization by the *Penicillium marneffei* RAC homolog. Journal of Cell Science. 2003;**116**(Pt 7):1249-1260

[41] Xi L, Xu X, Liu W, Li X, Liu Y, Li M, et al. Differentially expressed proteins of pathogenic *Penicillium marneffei* in yeast and mycelial phases. Journal of Medical Microbiology. 2007;**56**(Pt 3):298-304

[42] Rude TH, Toffaletti DL, Cox GM, Perfect JR. Relationship of the glyoxylate pathway to the pathogenesis of *Cryptococcus neoformans*. Infection and Immunity. 2002;**70**(10):5684-5694

[43] Derengowski LS, Tavares AH, Silva S, Procopio LS, Felipe MS, Silva-Pereira I. Upregulation of glyoxylate cycle genes

upon *Paracoccidioides brasiliensis* internalization by murine macrophages and *in vitro* nutritional stress condition. Medical Mycology. 2008;**46**(2):125-134

[44] Dunn MF, Ramirez-Trujillo JA, Hernandez-Lucas I. Major roles of isocitrate lyase and malate synthase in bacterial and fungal pathogenesis. Microbiology (Reading). 2009;**155**(Pt 10):3166-3175

[45] Fridovich I. Oxygen toxicity: A radical explanation. The Journal of Experimental Biology. 1998;**201**(Pt 8):1203-1209

[46] Missall TA, Lodge JK, McEwen JE. Mechanisms of resistance to oxidative and nitrosative stress: Implications for fungal survival in mammalian hosts. Eukaryotic Cell. 2004;**3**(4):835-846

[47] Shibuya K, Paris S, Ando T, Nakayama H, Hatori T, Latge JP. Catalases of *Aspergillus fumigatus* and inflammation in aspergillosis. Nihon Ishinkin Gakkai Zasshi. 2006;**47**(4):249-255

[48] Pongpom P, Cooper CR Jr, Vanittanakom N. Isolation and characterization of a catalase-peroxidase gene from the pathogenic fungus, *Penicillium marneffei*. Medical Mycology. 2005;**43**(5):403-411

[49] Pongpom M, Sawatdeechaikul P, Kummasook A, Khanthawong S, Vanittanakom N. Antioxidative and immunogenic properties of catalase-peroxidase protein in *Penicillium marneffei*. Medical Mycology. 2013;**51**(8):835-842

[50] Thirach S, Cooper CR Jr, Vanittanakom P, Vanittanakom N. The copper, zinc superoxide dismutase gene of *Penicillium marneffei*: Cloning, characterization, and differential expression during phase transition and macrophage infection. Medical Mycology. 2007;**45**(5):409-417

[51] Lindquist S, Craig EA. The heat-shock proteins. Annual Review of Genetics. 1988;**22**:631-677

[52] Kummasook A, Pongpom P, Vanittanakom N. Cloning, characterization and differential expression of an *hsp70* gene from the pathogenic dimorphic fungus,*Penicillium marneffei*. DNA Seqeuence. 2007;**18**(5):385-394

[53] Vanittanakom N, Pongpom M, Praparattanapan J, Cooper CR, Sirisanthana T. Isolation and expression of heat shock protein 30 gene from *Penicillium marneffei*. Medical Mycology. 2009;**47**(5):521-526

[54] Smith DFQ, Casadevall A. The role of melanin in fungal pathogenesis for animal hosts. Current Topics in Microbiology and Immunology. 2019;**422**:1-30

[55] Tsai HF, Wheeler MH, Chang YC, Kwon-Chung KJ. A developmentally regulated gene cluster involved in conidial pigment biosynthesis in *Aspergillus fumigatus*. Journal of Bacteriology. 1999;**181**(20):6469-6477

[56] Eisenman HC, Casadevall A. Synthesis and assembly of fungal melanin. Applied Microbiology and Biotechnology. 2012;**93**(3):931-940

[57] Woo PC, Lau CC, Chong KT, Tse H, Tsang DN, Lee RA, et al. MP1 homologue-based multilocus sequence system for typing the pathogenic fungus *Penicillium marneffei*: A novel approach using lineage-specific genes. Journal of Clinical Microbiology. 2007;**45**(11):3647-3654

[58] Tam EW, Tsang CC, Lau SK, Woo PC. Polyketides, toxins and pigments in

Penicillium marneffei. Toxins (Basel). 2015;7(11):4421-4436

[59] Sapmak A, Boyce KJ, Andrianopoulos A, Vanittanakom N. The *pbrB* gene encodes a laccase required for DHN-melanin synthesis in conidia of *Talaromyces (Penicillium) marneffei*. PLoS One. 2015;**10**(4):e0122728

[60] Youngchim S, Hay RJ, Hamilton AJ. Melanization of *Penicillium marneffei in vitro* and *in vivo*. Microbiology (Reading). 2005;**151**(Pt 1):291-299

[61] Liu D, Wei L, Guo T, Tan W. Detection of DOPA-melanin in the dimorphic fungal pathogen *Penicillium marneffei* and its effect on macrophage phagocytosis *in vitro*. PLoS One. 2014;**9**(3):e92610

[62] Wheeler MH, Bell AA. Melanins and their importance in pathogenic fungi. Current Topics in Medical Mycology. 1988;**2**:338-387

[63] Bull AT, Carter BL. The isolation of tyrosinase from *Aspergillus nidulans*, its kinetic and molecular properties and some consideration of its activity *in vivo*. Journal of General Microbiology. 1973;**75**(1):61-73

[64] Williamson PR. Biochemical and molecular characterization of the diphenol oxidase of *Cryptococcus neoformans*: Identification as a laccase. Journal of Bacteriology. 1994;**176**(3):656-664

[65] Liu S, Youngchim S, Zamith-Miranda D, Nosanchuk JD. Fungal melanin and the mammalian immune system. Journal of Fungi (Basel). 2021;7(4):264

[66] Cunha MM, Franzen AJ, Seabra SH, Herbst MH, Vugman NV, Borba LP, et al. Melanin in *Fonsecaea pedrosoi*: A trap for oxidative radicals. BMC Microbiology. 2010;**10**:80

[67] Volling K, Thywissen A, Brakhage AA, Saluz HP. Phagocytosis of melanized *Aspergillus* conidia by macrophages exerts cytoprotective effects by sustained PI3K/Akt signalling. Cellular Microbiology. 2011;**13**(8):1130-1148

[68] Chai LY, Netea MG, Sugui J, Vonk AG, van de Sande WW, Warris A, et al. *Aspergillus fumigatus* conidial melanin modulates host cytokine response. Immunobiology. 2010;**215**(11): 915-920

[69] Youngchim S. Melanization of Fungal Pathogens, Particularly *Aspergillus fumigatus* and *Penicillium marneffei*. London, UK: University of London; 2004

[70] Woo PC, Tam EW, Chong KT, Cai JJ, Tung ET, Ngan AH, et al. High diversity of polyketide synthase genes and the melanin biosynthesis gene cluster in *Penicillium marneffei*. The FEBS Journal. 2010;**277**(18):3750-3758

[71] Nosanchuk JD, Casadevall A. Impact of melanin on microbial virulence and clinical resistance to antimicrobial compounds. Antimicrobial Agents and Chemotherapy. 2006;**50**(11):3519-3528

[72] Ikeda F. Antifungal activity and clinical efficacy of micafungin sodium (Funguard). Nihon Yakurigaku Zasshi. 2003;**122**(4):339-344

[73] Kaewmalakul J, Nosanchuk JD, Vanittanakom N, Youngchim S. Melanization and morphological effects on antifungal susceptibility of *Penicillium marneffei*. Antonie Van Leeuwenhoek. 2014;**106**(5):1011-1020

[74] He X, Liu D, Chen Q. Proteomic analysis on the regulation of DOPA-melanin synthesis in *Talaromyces*

marneffei. Microbial Pathogenesis. 2021;**150**:104701

[75] Galhaup C, Goller S, Peterbauer CK, Strauss J, Haltrich D. Characterization of the major laccase isoenzyme from *Trametes pubescens* and regulation of its synthesis by metal ions. Microbiology (Reading). 2002;**148**(Pt 7):2159-2169

[76] Thurston C. The structure and function of fungal laccases. Micribiology. 1994;**140**:19-26

[77] SapmakA,KaewmalakulJ,NosanchukJD, Vanittanakom N, Andrianopoulos A, Pruksaphon K, et al. *Talaromyces marneffei* laccase modifies THP-1 macrophage responses. Virulence. 2016;**7**(6):702-717

[78] Douglas L. Adhesion of *Candida albicans* to host surface. FEMS Symposium. 1991;**50**:43-48

[79] Hearn V. Structure and function of the fungal cell wall. Fungal Disease. 1997:27-60

[80] Klis F. Review: Cell wall assembly in yeast. Yeast. 1994;**10**:851-869

[81] Shepherd MG, Gopal PK. Nature and control of cell wall biosynthesis. In: Bossche H, Odds FC, Kerridge D, editors. Dimorphic Fungi in Biology and Medicine. New York, NY: Springer; 1993. pp. 153-167

[82] Wong SS, Wong KH, Hui WT, Lee SS, Lo JY, Cao L, et al. Differences in clinical and laboratory diagnostic characteristics of penicilliosis marneffei in human immunodeficiency virus (HIV)- and non-HIV-infected patients. Journal of Clinical Microbiology. 2001;**39**(12):4535-4540

[83] Cao L, Chan CM, Lee C, Wong SS, Yuen KY. *MP1* encodes an abundant and highly antigenic cell wall mannoprotein in the pathogenic fungus *Penicillium marneffei*. Infection and Immunity. 1998;**66**(3):966-973

[84] Cao L, Chan KM, Chen D, Vanittanakom N, Lee C, Chan CM, et al. Detection of cell wall mannoprotein Mp1p in culture supernatants of *Penicillium marneffei* and in sera of penicilliosis patients. Journal of Clinical Microbiology. 1999;**37**(4):981-986

[85] Cao L, Chen DL, Lee C, Chan CM, Chan KM, Vanittanakom N, et al. Detection of specific antibodies to an antigenic mannoprotein for diagnosis of *Penicillium marneffei* penicilliosis. Journal of Clinical Microbiology. 1998;**36**(10):3028-3031

[86] Woo PC, Lau SK, Lau CC, Tung ET, Chong KT, Yang F, et al. Mp1p is a virulence factor in *Talaromyces (Penicillium) marneffei*. PLoS Neglected Tropical Diseases. 2016;**10**(8):e0004907

[87] Liao S, Tung ET, Zheng W, Chong K, Xu Y, Dai P, et al. Crystal structure of the Mp1p ligand binding domain 2 reveals its function as a fatty acid-binding protein. The Journal of Biological Chemistry. 2010;**285**(12):9211-9220

[88] Dennis EA, Norris PC. Eicosanoid storm in infection and inflammation. Nature Reviews. Immunology. 2015;**15**(8):511-523

[89] Lam WH, Sze KH, Ke Y, Tse MK, Zhang H, Woo PCY, et al. *Talaromyces marneffei* Mp1 protein, a novel virulence factor, carries two arachidonic acid-binding domains to suppress inflammatory responses in hosts. Infection and Immunity. 2019;**87**(4):e00679-e00618

[90] Park HS, Lee SC, Cardenas ME, Heitman J. Calcium-calmodulin-calcineurin signaling: A globally

conserved virulence cascade in eukaryotic microbial pathogens. Cell Host & Microbe. 2019;**26**(4):453-462

[91] Aramburu J, Rao A, Klee CB. Calcineurin: From structure to function. Current Topics in Cellular Regulation. 2000;**36**:237-295

[92] Rusnak F, Mertz P. Calcineurin: Form and function. Physiological Reviews. 2000;**80**(4):1483-1521

[93] Juvvadi PR, Lamoth F, Steinbach WJ. Calcineurin-mediated regulation of hyphal growth, septation, and virulence in *Aspergillus fumigatus*. Mycopathologia. 2014;**178**(5-6):341-348

[94] Juvvadi PR, Steinbach WJ. Calcineurin orchestrates hyphal growth, septation, drug resistance and pathogenesis of *Aspergillus fumigatus*: Where do we go from here? Pathogens. 2015;**4**(4):883-893

[95] Fu C, Donadio N, Cardenas ME, Heitman J. Dissecting the roles of the calcineurin pathway in unisexual reproduction, stress responses, and virulence in *Cryptococcus deneoformans*. Genetics. 2018;**208**(2):639-653

[96] Yu SJ, Chang YL, Chen YL. Calcineurin signaling: Lessons from *Candida* species. FEMS Yeast Research. 2015;**15**(4):fov016

[97] Chen YL, Konieczka JH, Springer DJ, Bowen SE, Zhang J, Silao FG, et al. Convergent evolution of calcineurin pathway roles in thermotolerance and virulence in *Candida glabrata*., G3 (Bethesda). 2012;**2**(6):675-691

[98] Chen YL, Yu SJ, Huang HY, Chang YL, Lehman VN, Silao FG, et al. Calcineurin controls hyphal growth, virulence, and drug tolerance of *Candida tropicalis*. Eukaryotic Cell. 2014;**13**(7):844-854

[99] Campos CB, Di Benedette JP, Morais FV, Ovalle R, Nobrega MP. Evidence for the role of calcineurin in morphogenesis and calcium homeostasis during mycelium-to-yeast dimorphism of *Paracoccidioides brasiliensis*. Eukaryotic Cell. 2008;**7**(10):1856-1864

[100] Zheng YQ, Pan KS, Latge JP, Andrianopoulos A, Luo H, Yan RF, et al. Calcineurin A is essential in the regulation of asexual development, stress responses and pathogenesis in *Talaromyces marneffei*. Frontiers in Microbiology. 2019;**10**:3094

[101] Douglas CM, D'Ippolito JA, Shei GJ, Meinz M, Onishi J, Marrinan JA, et al. Identification of the FKS1 gene of *Candida albicans* as the essential target of 1,3-beta-D-glucan synthase inhibitors. Antimicrobial Agents and Chemotherapy. 1997;**41**(11):2471-2479

[102] Coffey R, Ganz T. Iron homeostasis: An anthropocentric perspective. The Journal of Biological Chemistry. 2017;**292**(31):12727-12734

[103] Nairz M, Weiss G. Iron in infection and immunity. Molecular Aspects of Medicine. 2020;**75**:100864

[104] Taramelli D, Brambilla S, Sala G, Bruccoleri A, Tognazioli C, Riviera-Uzielli L, et al. Effects of iron on extracellular and intracellular growth of *Penicillium marneffei*. Infection and Immunity. 2000;**68**(3):1724-1726

[105] Johnson L. Iron and siderophores in fungal-host interactions. Mycological Research. 2008;**112**(Pt 2):170-183

[106] Kosman DJ. Molecular mechanisms of iron uptake in fungi. Molecular Microbiology. 2003;**47**(5):1185-1197

[107] Kosman DJ. Redox cycling in iron uptake, efflux, and trafficking.

The Journal of Biological Chemistry. 2010;**285**(35):26729-26735

[108] Pasricha S, Payne M, Canovas D, Pase L, Ngaosuwankul N, Beard S, et al. Cell-type-specific transcriptional profiles of the dimorphic pathogen *Penicillium marneffei* reflect distinct reproductive, morphological, and environmental demands. G3 (Bethesda). 2013;**3**(11):1997-2014

[109] Pasricha S, Schafferer L, Lindner H, Joanne Boyce K, Haas H, Andrianopoulos A. Differentially regulated high-affinity iron assimilation systems support growth of the various cell types in the dimorphic pathogen *Talaromyces marneffei*. Molecular Microbiology. 2016;**102**(4):715-737

[110] Pongpom M, Amsri A, Sukantamala P, Suwannaphong P, Jeenkeawpieam J. Expression of *Talaromyces marneffei acuM* and *acuK* genes in gluconeogenic substrates and various iron concentrations. Journal of Fungi (Basel). 2020;**6**(3):102

[111] Suzuki Y, Murray SL, Wong KH, Davis MA, Hynes MJ. Reprogramming of carbon metabolism by the transcriptional activators *AcuK* and *AcuM* in *Aspergillus nidulans*. Molecular Microbiology. 2012;**84**(5):942-964

[112] Pongpom M, Liu H, Xu W, Snarr BD, Sheppard DC, Mitchell AP, et al. Divergent targets of *Aspergillus fumigatus AcuK* and *AcuM* transcription factors during growth *in vitro* versus invasive disease. Infection and Immunity. 2015;**83**(3):923-933

[113] Amsri A, Jeenkeawpieam J, Sukantamala P, Pongpom M. Role of *acuK* in control of iron acquisition and gluconeogenesis in *Talaromyces marneffei*. Journal of Fungi (Basel). 2021;**7**(10):798

[114] Rodrigues ML, Nakayasu ES, Oliveira DL, Nimrichter L, Nosanchuk JD, Almeida IC, et al. Extracellular vesicles produced by *Cryptococcus neoformans* contain protein components associated with virulence. Eukaryotic Cell. 2008;**7**(1):58-67

[115] Rodrigues ML, Nakayasu ES, Almeida IC, Nimrichter L. The impact of proteomics on the understanding of functions and biogenesis of fungal extracellular vesicles. Journal of Proteomics. 2014;**97**:177-186

[116] Oliveira DL, Rizzo J, Joffe LS, Godinho RM, Rodrigues ML. Where do they come from and where do they go: Candidates for regulating extracellular vesicle formation in fungi. International Journal of Molecular Sciences. 2013;**14**(5):9581-9603

[117] Vallejo MC, Nakayasu ES, Matsuo AL, Sobreira TJ, Longo LV, Ganiko L, et al. Vesicle and vesicle-free extracellular proteome of *Paracoccidioides brasiliensis*: Comparative analysis with other pathogenic fungi. Journal of Proteome Research. 2012;**11**(3):1676-1685

[118] Vargas G, Rocha JD, Oliveira DL, Albuquerque PC, Frases S, Santos SS, et al. Compositional and immunobiological analyses of extracellular vesicles released by *Candida albicans*. Cellular Microbiology. 2015;**17**(3):389-407

[119] Alves LR, Peres da Silva R, Sanchez DA, Zamith-Miranda D, Rodrigues ML, Goldenberg S, et al. Extracellular vesicle-mediated RNA release in *Histoplasma capsulatum*. mSphere. 2019;**4**(2):e00176-e00119

[120] Yang B, Wang J, Jiang H, Lin H, Ou Z, Ullah A, et al. Extracellular vesicles derived from *Talaromyces marneffei* yeasts mediate inflammatory response in macrophage cells by bioactive protein

components. Frontiers in Microbiology. 2020;**11**:603183

[121] Drouhet E. Penicilliosis due to *Penicillium marneffei*: A new emerging systemic mycosis in AIDS patients travelling or living in Southeast Asia. Journal of Mycological Médicine (Paris). 1993;**4**:195-224

[122] Supparatpinyo K, Chiewchanvit S, Hirunsri P, Uthammachai C, Nelson KE, Sirisanthana T. *Penicillium marneffei* infection in patients infected with human immunodeficiency virus. Clinical Infectious Diseases. 1992;**14**(4):871-874

[123] Wang YF, Cai JP, Wang YD, Dong H, Hao W, Jiang LX, et al. Immunoassays based on *Penicillium marneffei* Mp1p derived from Pichia pastoris expression system for diagnosis of penicilliosis. PLoS One. 2011;**6**(12):e28796

[124] Thu NTM, Chan JFW, Ly VT, Ngo HT, Hien HTA, Lan NPH, et al. Superiority of a novel Mp1p antigen detection enzyme immunoassay compared to standard BACTEC blood culture in the diagnosis of Talaromycosis. Clinical Infectious Diseases. 2021;**73**(2):e330-e336

[125] Wang YF, Xu HF, Han ZG, Zeng L, Liang CY, Chen XJ, et al. Serological surveillance for *Penicillium marneffei* infection in HIV-infected patients during 2004-2011 in Guangzhou, China. Clinical Microbiology Infections. 2015;**21**(5):484-489

[126] Pickering JW, Sant HW, Bowles CA, Roberts WL, Woods GL. Evaluation of a (1->3)-beta-D-glucan assay for diagnosis of invasive fungal infections. Journal of Clinical Microbiology. 2005;**43**(12):5957-5962

[127] Kozel TR, Bauman SK. CrAg lateral flow assay for cryptococcosis. Expert Opinion in Medical Diagnostic. 2012;**6**(3):245-251

[128] Krajaejun T, Imkhieo S, Intaramat A, Ratanabanangkoon K. Development of an immunochromatographic test for rapid serodiagnosis of human pythiosis. Clinical and Vaccine Immunology. 2009;**16**(4):506-509

[129] Marot-Leblond A, Grimaud L, David S, Sullivan DJ, Coleman DC, Ponton J, et al. Evaluation of a rapid immunochromatographic assay for identification of *Candida albicans* and *Candida dubliniensis*. Journal of Clinical Microbiology. 2004;**42**(11):4956-4960

[130] Thornton CR. Development of an immunochromatographic lateral-flow device for rapid serodiagnosis of invasive aspergillosis. Clinical and Vaccine Immunology. 2008;**15**(7):1095-1105

[131] Chastain DB, Henao-Martinez AF, Franco-Paredes C. Opportunistic invasive mycoses in AIDS: Cryptococcosis, Histoplasmosis, Coccidiodomycosis, and Talaromycosis. Current Infectious Disease Reports. 2017;**19**(10):36

[132] Pruksaphon K, Intaramat A, Ratanabanangkoon K, Nosanchuk JD, VanittanakomN,YoungchimS.Development and characterization of an immunochromatographic test for the rapid diagnosis of *Talaromyces (Penicillium) marneffei*. PLoS One. 2018;**13**(4):e0195596

[133] Pruksaphon K, Intaramat A, Simsiriwong P, Mongkolsuk S, Ratanabanangkoon K, Nosanchuk JD, et al. An inexpensive point-of-care immunochromatographic test for *Talaromyces marneffei* infection based on the yeast phase specific monoclonal antibody 4D1 and *Galanthus nivalis* agglutinin. PLoS Neglected Tropical Diseases. 2021;**15**(5):e0009058

[134] LoBuglio KF, Taylor JW. Phylogeny and PCR identification of the human pathogenic fungus *Penicillium marneffei*. Journal of Clinical Microbiology. 1995;**33**(1):85-89

[135] Vanittanakom N, Merz WG, Sittisombut N, Khamwan C, Nelson KE, Sirisanthana T. Specific identification of *Penicillium marneffei* by a polymerase chain reaction/hybridization technique. Medical Mycology. 1998;**36**(3):169-175

[136] Prariyachatigul C, Chaiprasert A, Geenkajorn K, Kappe R, Chuchottaworn C, Termsetjaroen S, et al. Development and evaluation of a one-tube seminested PCR assay for the detection and identification of *Penicillium marneffei*. Mycoses. 2003;**46**(11-12):447-454

[137] Lu S, Li X, Calderone R, Zhang J, Ma J, Cai W, et al. Whole blood nested PCR and real-time PCR amplification of *Talaromyces marneffei* specific DNA for diagnosis. Medical Mycology. 2016;**54**(2):162-168

[138] Zhang J, Zhang D, Du J, Zhou Y, Cai Y, Sun R, et al. Rapid diagnosis of *Talaromyces marneffei* infection assisted by metagenomic next-generation sequencing in a HIV-negative patient. IDCases. 2021;**23**:e01055

[139] Zhang W, Ye J, Qiu C, Wang L, Jin W, Jiang C, et al. Rapid and precise diagnosis of *T. marneffei* pulmonary infection in a HIV-negative patient with autosomal-dominant *STAT3* mutation: A case report. Therapeutic Advances in Respiratory Diseases. 2020;**14**:175

Chapter 4

Evolution of Parasitism and Pathogenic Adaptations in Certain Medically Important Fungi

Gokul Shankar Sabesan, Ranjit Singh Aja, Ranjith Mehenderkar and Basanta Kumar Mohanty

Abstract

Fungi are eukaryotes designated as a separate kingdom because of their unique characteristics different from both animals and plants. Fungi are mainly classified into two major types as "saprobes" and "parasites" depending on their type of nutrition and existence. It is postulated that the present-day parasites also once existed as saprophytes in the soil. It is also curious to find the reasons on what early events could have been responsible for the evolution of the saprobes into human parasites? During this process of evolution, some of the anthropophilic organisms have totally lost all their soil-inhabiting traits and the ability for saprophytic survival, while few others have successfully retained their ability to survive in two different ecological niches (soil and animal/human host). The various possible reasons, such as predation, antagonism, and other factors contributing to the emergence of parasitic adaptations, are discussed using examples of dermatophytes, *Cryptococcus neoformans,* and *Histoplasma capsulatum.*

Keywords: fungal parasitism, fungal virulence factors, adaptations, fungal evolution, *Cryptococcus neoformans*, *Histoplasma capsulatum*, dermatophytes, dimorphism, anthropophization, fungal pathogenesis

1. Introduction

Fungi are a group of eukaryotic organisms existing in the ecosystem as chemoheterotrophs, as they are dependent mostly upon the secretary exoenzymes to harvest energy from the organic substrates. Based on the heterotrophic nutrition and their dependency for survival, fungi are mainly classified into two major types: (a) saprobes and (b) parasites. Interestingly, there is difficulty to have a clear distinction between the human parasites and saprophytes as the natural habitats of most of these pathogenic fungi that cause systemic mycoses are only the dead and decaying organic matter. These fungi mostly dwell in soils enriched by droppings of birds or other organic wastes. Fungal parasitism is considered to be one of the largest areas in medical mycology that has attracted so many researchers all over the globe over the years. Enormous research work had been carried out in plant-parasitic fungi, but the role of fungi in veterinary and human medicine until recent years remained the

IntechOpen

most neglected area, the reason being that most of the medically important fungi are opportunistic pathogens and that the person-to-person transmission of fungal diseases is not as common as the bacterial/viral infections.

In recent years, fungal diseases have reached epidemic proportions in causing morbidity and mortality all over the world as it is regarded that it may be just the tip of the iceberg. Increasing immunocompromised status in human beings due to the advent of human immunodeficiency virus/AIDS, chemotherapy, radiotherapy, debilitating illness such as cancer, COVID-19, prolonged steroid treatment, organ transplantation, and chronic diseases perhaps are the conditions that would have promoted these opportunistic pathogenic fungi into "Champion parasites" in causing human diseases [1]. Thus, these so-called low virulent saprophytic fungi are capable of causing diseases given the opportunity and availability of susceptible hosts. It is always of immense interest and curiosity to know why these fungi would have adapted themselves or equipped to develop virulence factors to emerge as human pathogens/parasites. It would always be necessary to understand what early events or environmental factors in their original habitats would have compelled/prompted/facilitated certain groups of soil-inhabiting fungi to emerge as human pathogens [2].

2. Fungal parasitism

Fungi exhibit three types of parasitism [3] in human beings:

1. Obligate parasitism as seen in the case of certain anthropophilic dermatophytes and *Malassezia* species.

2. Parasitism to the extent of true pathogenesis as seen in the case of dimorphic systemic fungi, viz., *Histoplasma capsulatum, Blastomyces dermatitidis, Coccidioides immitis,* and *Paracoccidioides brasiliensis.*

3. Parasitism is an accidental/opportunistic event, as seen in the case of *C. neoformans* and *Candida* species.

3. Obligate parasitism

Obligate parasitism is seen in the case of anthropophilic dermatophytes, such as *Trichophyton rubrum, Trichophyton mentagrophytes, Trichophyton tonsurans, Trichophyton violaceum*, and *Epidermophyton floccosum* [4]. It is also seen in the case of the lipophilic yeast, *Malassezia species*, viz., *Malassezia furfur and Malassezia globosa.* The existence of these organisms in "ex-anthropophilic" conditions for a prolonged period has not been established yet [5]. Several experimental studies [5] conducted on the saprophytic survivability of these organisms in the soil also reveal that these organisms, if at all, can exist in the soil only for a transient period. However, their counterparts, related groups of dermatophytes such as *Nannizzia gypsea* (previously named *Microsporum gypseum*), *Microsporum nanum, Microsporum distortum,* and *Trichophyton ajelloi*, can exist in soil popularly as the geophilic group. Interestingly, the genetic variation between the anthropophilic and geophilic groups of dermatophytes is calculated less.

The possible theory [3, 6] by which certain dermatophytes would have evolved as obligate parasites in human beings would have started and progressed in different phases.

1. Geophilism of these fungi in the burrows of smaller mammals.

2. Colonization of the hair/fur of these small mammals.

3. Parasitism in these mammals leads to synanthropophization

4. Well-established anthropophization as seen in the case of *T. rubrum* by losing all the geophilic characteristics, such as conidial abundance and ornamentation, osmotolerance, heterothallic mating, etc. [4].

Although the above theory clearly suggests the means of the development of parasitism in dermatophytes, it drastically fails to explain why it had occurred in certain species of dermatophytes. Furthermore, what was the sequence of events that occurred in their original habitat that would have compelled/promoted these fungi to become obligate pathogens beg an answer. Furthermore, it is also important to understand how these organisms adapt themselves to lead an obligate anthropophilic existence. In *Malassezia* spp., a similar lineage is seen, as the members of the species exist only as obligate parasites (commensals) in animals. There are no reports of the existence of *Malassezia* spp. in the soil so far.

4. Parasitism and true pathogenesis

In the case of obligate parasitic fungi, such as *T. rubrum*, their existence is exclusively limited to the human habitat; hence, the diseases caused by these organisms are not debilitating or life-threatening, whereas parasitism is truly severe in true pathogenic fungi, such *as C. immitis, H. capsulatum, P. brasiliensis*, and *B. dermatitidis.* These systemic dimorphic fungi exist as saprophytes in the soil, droppings/guano of bats, and pellets of various avifauna, but these organisms accidentally encounter the human habitat. They exhibit true pathogenic potential even in the immunocompetent host. This ability to cause life-threatening infections irrespective of the immune status of the host is intriguing, and it is really amazing to know how these fungi evolved the super specialty of existing in the saprophytic form and yet cause diseases in "immunocompetent" people. The dimorphic mode of existence of these fungi is largely considered to be one of the predominant selective advantages [7] for their successful geophilism and anthropophization. One of the most intriguing aspects of its biology is the dimorphism exhibited by *H. capsulatum. H. capsulatum* produces mycelium at environmental temperatures less than 30°C, but reproduces as a budding yeast when growing intracellularly in patients with histoplasmosis. It has been estimated that in the endemic areas of the United States (histoplasmosis surveillance data of 2011–2014), the average incidence all over the country ranges even up to 39 cases per 100,000 population [8]. Though histoplasmosis is endemic to certain places and limited to certain geographical locations, *H. capsulatum* is found throughout the world [3].

5. Opportunistic parasitism

Opportunistic pathogens are fungi that strike and cause infections under certain predisposing host conditions, such as severe immunodeficiency. These fungi are also widely present in soil bird droppings as saprophytes. When a host is available in an immunocompromised state, these fungi cause moderate to life-threatening diseases, as seen in the case of cryptococcal meningitis caused by *C. neoformans*. Several studies have shown that cryptococcal infection poses a major threat to the life of AIDS patients and other immunocompromised people all over the world. It would be interesting to unknot the mystery of how *Cryptococcus* species, originally a geophilic saprophytic yeast, can "spontaneously specialize" by developing several mechanisms/virulence factors to invade, colonize, and manifest life-threatening disease in the human host.

Serious uncertainties exist in finding plausible answers to these questions:

a. Whether the lack of immune barrier in the host is the prime cause to elicit an infection (or)

b. The gradual development of parasitic adaptations in the course of evolution of *Cryptococcus* species have contributed to the parasitism?

c. Is there a changing face of this pathogen in the course of evolution? (opportunistic to truly pathogenic)

d. The adaptations to the parasitic life, which include the production of pigment (melanin), mannitol utilization, urease activity, and encapsulation in *C. neoformans* are unique and are seen only in certain fungi among the whole of the geophilic community. Do these characters provide an advantage for survival in the ecological niche for this pathogen?

e. Is the organism exhibiting a growing ecological niche with more and more newer habitats or reservoirs (droppings in different avifauna such as crows, water birds, etc.)

f. Better elucidation of such uniqueness in *Cryptococcus* species is essential for developing a better management strategy for fungal diseases.

For practical purposes, in the realm of Medical Mycology, the infectious microorganisms have been grouped into three ecological categories based on their natural histories. These entities, in a broad sense, have been traditionally designated as being geophilic, zoophilic, and anthropophilic and are designed as follows:

1. **Geophilic**: Free living organisms that exist as saprobes in soil subsisting on dead organic matter.

2. **Zoophilic**: Organisms that cannot constitutionally exist in soil as saprobes but evolved to live primarily on or in the bodies of animals other than humans.

3. **Anthropophilic**: Organisms that are unable to survive as free-living entities in soil but have evolved to be components of the microbiota of humans.

Interestingly, some geophilic and zoophilic organisms also cause human infections.

It is also curious to find the reasons for what early events could have been responsible for the evolution of the "Saprobes" into human "Parasites"? The line of demarcation between the saprophytes and parasites is neither here nor there.

6. Fungal evolution: pathogens and their parasitic adaptations

Organism	Virulence factors	Environmental advantage	Survival in Host/ adaptability	Parasitic adaptation
C. neoformans	Capsule	Escape phagocytosis of amoebae	Escape phagocytosis by macrophages	Important virulence factors in human infection
	Melanin	Protection from Sunlight/UV Escape predation from soil macroorganisms	Resistance to antifungals Shield against immunologically active cells.	Able to use DOPA in CNS to cause meningitis
	Urease	Unknown. May contribute to the nutritional role in nitrogen acquisition.	Promotes nonlytic exocytosis	Survival advantage in a human host
	Phospholipase	Unknown	*C. neoformans*, calcineurin responds to stress caused by cell-wall-perturbing agents, physiological temperature of host, alkaline pH, high CO_2, and high cation concentration [9]	Calcineurin activation is essential for a. virulence and b. hyphal elongation during sexual reproduction (mating and monokaryotic fruiting) [9]
H. capsulatum	Ornamentation Tuberculate macroconidia	May protect against predation by soil macroflora (mites, earthworms)	—	Spores disseminated by wind are inhaled
	Dimorphism	Survive as a mold at 25°C	Intracellular survival as yeast at 37°C Resistance to microbiocidal products of neutrophils	Mold-to-yeast conversion is an important aspect of pathogenesis (similar phenomenon in other true pathogenic fungi *B. dermatitidis, C. immitis* and *P. brasiliensis*).
Dermatophytes	Keratinase, collagenases	Nutrition (utilize keratin from dead animal issues)	Degrades scleroproteins in skin, hair, and nail	
	Elastase	Nutrition (utilize keratin from dead animal issues)	Degrades elastin, scleroproteins	Enhances invasion of elastin containing tissue
	Pigment production		Resistance to antifungals.	Identification tool in diagnostic mycology
	Obligate parasitism	Loss of saprophytic survivability and soil association characteristics in certain anthropophilic dermatophytes	Enzyme moderation (protease). Loss of hair perforation ability, enzymes (such as urease), osmotolerance, etc. Exhibit slow growth rate.	Cause mild and chronic infections

Organism	Virulence factors	Environmental advantage	Survival in Host/ adaptability	Parasitic adaptation
Candida species	Cell wall glycoproteins	—	Adherence to epithelial surfaces	
	Acid protease	—	Cleavage of IgA2	
	Morphological variation Ability to switch reversibly into different colony types at high frequencies.	—	Allows organisms to adapt to a different environment in the host.	Colonies of varying nature (smooth, rough, hat, fuzzy wrinkle, star, and stippled)
	Phospholipases	—	Hydrolyze ester linkages of glycophospholipids	
	Secretory aspartic proteinases	—	Promote adherence and survival of the pathogen on mucosal surfaces.	Facilitate invasion of host tissues
	Biofilming	—	Resistance to antifungals	
	Dimorphism	—	Ability to form hyphae helps in tissue invasion	

7. Antibiosis by other soil fungi

It has long been speculated and later had been confirmed using modern phylogenetic studies that the parasitic dermatophytes probably arose from the geophilic (soil-borne) nonpathogenic ancestors. The existence of today's nonpathogenic dermatophytoids in the same habitat is the exemplification for this hypothesis (e.g., *T. ajelloi* and *Trichophyton terrestre*) [10–12].

The studies by Gokulshankar et al. [13] revealed that the Secretory substances (SS) released by *Chrysosporium keratinophillum* possess significant inhibitory (antidermatophytic) activity against *T. tonsurans*, *T. rubrum*, *T. violaceum*, *T. mentagrophytes*, and *E. floccosum*. The SS of *C. keratinophillum* released on the 15th day inhibited all the isolates of *T. rubrum*, while the SS released on the 10th day inhibited all the isolates of *T. tonsurans*, *T. violaceum*, and *E. floccosum* [13].

The Secretory substances of *C. keratinophillum* further failed to inhibit the growth of the geophilic *N. gypsea* (previously named *M. gypseum*) and zoophilic *Microsporum canis*. This experiment should be correlated with the global prevalence of *N. gypsea* in soil. The selective ability of *N. gypsea* to counter the antagonistic activity of the SS of *C. keratinophillum* may be one of the reasons for the worldwide distribution of this fungus in soil [14].

It is also interesting to note that in the co-inoculation studies, when *C. keratinophillum* and anthropophilic dermatophytes were co-inoculated on Sabouraud Dextrose Agar (SDA), *C. keratinophillum* failed to inhibit the mycelial growth of *T. ton*surans, *T. rubrum*, *T. mentagrophytes*, and *E. floccosum*. However, conidia formation did not occur on the organisms (*T. rubrum*, *T. tonsurans,* and *E. floccosum)* when they were grown near *C. keratinophillum*. It is presumed that (a) the nature and (b) the quantity of the SS released by *C. keratinophillum* may affect the growth of these pathogenic dermatophytes. It may be because the SS produced by *C. keratinophillum* during its early growth phase might not be very active to inhibit. Furthermore, when both *C. keratinophillum* and an anthropophilic species of dermatophytes were co-inoculated at the same time, the growth of dermatophytes may also start much before the actual release of SS (10–15 days) by *C. keratinophillum*. The absence of conidia formation in *E. floccosum, T. rubrum,* and *T. tonsurans* when grown near the *C. keratinophillum* establishes the fact that SS of this organism possesses definite antidermatophytic characteristics.

Gokulshankar et al. [14] and Gokulshankar et al. [13] performed co-inoculation studies of different individual species of pathogenic dermatophytes along with *C. keratinophillum* in both sterilized and unsterilized soil to study their compatibility in the near natural environment. Recovery of the dermatophytes was attempted at different time intervals. The results showed that none of the anthropophilic dermatophytes could be recovered after 15 days of incubation by either plating or hair baiting techniques. However, the dermatophytes could be recovered up to 40 days from sterilized soil when inoculated alone.

Interestingly, the isolation of geophilic *N. gypsea* (previously named *M. gypseum*) was not affected in these co-inoculation studies. The authors also found that whenever the baiting technique is employed for the isolation of dermatophytes from the soil, *Chrysosporium* species are the predominant fungi to be isolated [14]. *Chrysosporium* and allied genera accounted for 53.8% distribution, with *C. indicum* being the dominant species among the keratinophilic fungi in soil [15]. The attribution of *Chrysosporium* spp. as a principal contributor to the evolutionary divergence of some geophilic archi-dermatophyte to obligate parasitic dermatophyte species, such as *T rubrum and E. floccosum* [13].

The antibiosis of other soil-inhabiting microbes (bacteria, protozoans, etc.) on dermatophytes also cannot be ruled out or underestimated for their probable role in the evolution of parasitism in anthropophilic dermatophytes. Gokulshankar [16] tested several other soil-inhabiting fungi, such as *Aspergillus fumigatus, Aspergillus niger, Aspergillus flavus, Rhizopus oryzae*, *Penicillium sp,* and *Curvularia lunata* for antidermatophyte activity. Among the tested fungi, the SS and intracellular substances (ICS) of *C. lunata* were found to have a definite role in inhibition.

It was reported that *C. keratinophillum, A. flavus, A. niger, A. fumigatus, R. oryzae, Penicillium sp,* and *C. lunata* showed inhibitory effects on the lipophilic fungus, *M. furfur* on co-inoculation. Furthermore, the ICS and SS of *C. keratinophillum, A. flavus, A. niger, A. fumigatus, R. oryzae, Penicillium sp,* and *C. lunata* tested were also found to inhibit *M. furfur*. This clearly proves *M. furfur's* inability to co-exist with any of the tested environmentally prevalent fungi. Furthermore, *Malassezia* species are found only as obligate commensal/parasite on the human and/or animal hosts. The saprophytic existence of *M. furfur* or any other species of *Malassezia* is also not known. All these correlations helped Gokulshankar et al. [2] to contemplate and propose a hypothesis

i. Did the inhibition by the soil/environmentally prevalent fungi forced *M. furfur* to adapt to an obligate parasitic/commensal existence?

ii. Can this inhibition be considered as one of the early events in the course of evolution?? (But this hypothesis holds good if only there had been a past survival (existence) of *Malassezia* species or their related ancestors in soil).

The study has been done only with *C. keratinophillum,* but the possible role of other species of *Chrysosporium* group could have also contributed to the evolution process.

Several other environmental factors in combination with the antagonism/inhibition of other soil protozoa/fungi/bacteria could have compelled the dermatophytes to evolve parasitic adaptations. The reported low incidence of the anthropophilic dermatophytes in soil may also be due to the gradual weaning off soil-inhabiting characters (well-defined anthropophization) in these pathogenic dermatophytes.

8. Saprophytic survivability of obligate parasitic dermatophytes in soil

Several studies suggest that saprophytic survivability for parasitic dermatophytes in soil may not be possible due to their well-defined anthropophization. However, the viability of the fungal elements (chlamydospores and arthroconidia) in soil for a shorter period cannot be ruled out. Likewise, the recovery of *M. canis,* a zoophilic dermatophyte, even from sterile soil by either hair baiting or plating technique was also not possible after 60 days, which suggested that this organism is not capable of soil existence. Did the organism lose the ability to survive even as a spore in soil for a prolonged period?

The recovery of *N. gypsea* (previously named *M. gypseum*) was possible from both unsterile and sterile soil for up to 120 days. The recovery was possible by hair bating and plating methods, substantiating the saprophytic surviving ability of *N. gypsea* [13, 14, 16].

Hair baiting was found to be a superior method for isolating all keratinophilic fungi from soil, especially the dermatophytes. The study suggests that saprophytic survival even without the interference of other micro- or macroorganisms may not be possible for the obligate anthropophilic dermatophytes, such as *E. floccosum, T. tonsurans, T. rubrum,* and *T. violaceum* (**Tables 1** and **2**).

Test organisms	Number of isolates	Recovery in days/number of isolates							
		10	20	30	40	50	60	90	120
T. rubrum	4	2+	—	—	—	—	—	—	—
T. mentagrophytes	4	2+	1+	—	—	—	—	—	—
T. tonsurans	4	—	—	—	—	—	—	—	—
T. violaceum	4	—	—	—	—	—	—	—	—
E. floccosum	4	—	—	—	—	—	—	—	—
N. gypsea	4	4+	4+	4+	4+	4+	4+	4+	4+
M. canis	4	4+	4+	3+	—	—	—	—	—

Note: + could be recovered, – could not be recovered.

Table 1.
Saprophytic survivability of test organisms in unsterile soil by hair baiting technique.

Test organisms	Number of isolates	Recovery in days/number of isolates							
		10	20	30	40	50	60	90	120
T. rubrum	4	2+	—	—	—	—	—	—	—
T. mentagrophytes	4	2+	1+	—	—	—	—	—	—
T. tonsurans	4	—	—	—	—	—	—	—	—
T. violaceum	4	—	—	—	—	—	—	—	—

Test organisms	Number of isolates	Recovery in days/number of isolates							
		10	20	30	40	50	60	90	120
E. floccosum	4	—	—	—	—	—	—	—	—
N. gypsea	4	4+	4+	4+	4+	4+	4+	4+	4+
M. canis	4	4+	4+	2+	—	—	—	—	—
M. furfur	4	—	—	—	—	—	—	—	—
C. neoformans	4	2+	—	—	—	—	—	—	—
H. capsulatum-Yeast form	2	—	—	—	—	—	—	—	—
H. capsulatum-Mold form	2	2+	2+	2+	2+	2+	2+	2+	2+

Note: + could be recovered, – could not be recovered.

Table 2.
Saprophytic survivability of test organisms in unsterile soil by a soil plating technique.

9. Earthworms as predators of anthropophilic dermatophytes and *M. furfur*

Results of the feeding studies of earthworms with dermatophytes [17] have revealed that either the anthropophilic (*T. rubrum, T. mentagrophytes, T. tonsurans, T. violaceum*, and *E. floccosum)* or zoophilic dermatophyte species (*M. canis*) were unable to survive in the gut of the earthworm. The recovery in culture from the gut of earthworms or the worm cast was not possible. However, all the species were recovered from control plates in the absence of earthworms (plates containing just soil admixed with milk powder and egg). This experiment portrayed that the earthworm gut may not be an ideal environment for the survival of these parasitic dermatophytes. However, all the tested strains of *N. gypsea* were recovered from the gut and the worm cast.

Four earthworm species were used in the study (*Amynthas alexandri, Lampito mauritii, Aporrectodea tuberculate,* and *Lumbricus terrestris*). The gut extracts of all the four species of earthworms showed a similar band pattern at the retention factor in Thin layer Chromatography (Rf) value of 0.32. This pattern probably may represent some inhibiting enzymes/antidermatophytic factors.

Further recovery of *M. furfur* from the gut of earthworms/worm cast after feeding assay with earthworms was also not possible.

10. Saprophytic existence of *C. neoformans* and *H. capsulatum* in soil

Saprophytic survival of *C. neoformans* was recorded in sterile soil for up to 120 days, but it was not possible in unsterile soil. Steenbergen and Casadevall [18] and others have reported predation of *C. neoformans* by soil organisms such as nematodes and amoebae, as reported by earlier workers. The soil predators would have been eliminated in the process of sterilization, which could be the reason for their survival and recovery in sterile soil, whereas their survivability was affected in unsterile soil. Interestingly, both the melanin-producing and non-melanin-producing isolates could be isolated from sterile soil.

Saprophytic survivability for *H. capsulatum* was reported for up to 120 days only for the mold suspension of the organism. However, the yeast suspension could not survive both in sterile and unsterile soil (10–20 days). This clearly illustrates that yeast morphogenesis is an important adaptation developed by the *C. neoformans,* which is required for survival in the host (for pathogenic intracellular state), while the mold form is mandatory for the existence in soil as saprophyte (**Table 2**).

11. Protease moderation in dermatophytes and pathogenesis

The roles of protease in the pathogenesis of many microorganisms have been described [19]. Associations of protease in infections caused by *Candida* spp. and *Pseudomonas aeruginosa* have been documented [20, 21]. For the hydrolysis of structural proteins of skin, hair, and nails, dermatophytes require and, therefore, elaborate certain protein hydrolyzing enzymes. Lu [22] has reported that the hair perforation of *T. mentagrophytes* was due to certain enzymes. The roles of these enzymes in the pathogenesis of the disease have been established [23].

High enzyme activity was seen during the vegetative growth phase of all the species of anthropophilic dermatophytes studied. The enzyme activity of *N. gypsea* (previously named *M. gypseum*) and *M. canis* was found to be high during both the vegetative and sporulation phases by Ranganathan et al. [24]. Zoophilic and geophilic species usually evoke a severe inflammatory response in humans [25] on infection and is almost and always severe. Whether the ability to produce high levels of protease during the sporulation phase by *N. gypsea* and *M. canis* is the cause of the severe nature of infection when they clinically manifest in their unusual host (man) warrants a detailed study. However, a possible correlation between the abilities to produce high levels of proteolytic enzymes during both sporulation and vegetative phases of growth to the severity of infection may not be ruled out. The lowest enzyme activity among the anthropophilic group was recorded in all the strains of *T. rubrum* during the sporulation phase compared to the vegetative growth phase in all the isolates. Rippon [3] has reported enhanced sporulation during parasitism. The low level of enzyme production during sporulation in *T. rubrum* might be the reason for the mild lesions produced in the host. The severity of the lesions produced by *T. rubrum* is less compared to other dermatophytes species. As Gokulshankar [16] reported, it is strikingly evident that all the clinical isolates of *T. rubrum* were from chronic cases, and the case history of three isolates indicates the persistence of lesions for more than two years. In general, it is understandable that the noninflammatory mild lesions would be neglected by the patients and, therefore, are untreated. Rippon [3] also noted that the protease production is highly host specific, and the organism showed reduced physiological activity when growing on their preferred host (animal/man). This is a clear exemplification of the well-established anthropophization of the parasitic dermatophyte species.

The medium used to study the enzyme activity during sporulation was Takashio broth (1/10 diluted Sabouraud's dextrose broth with KH_2PO_4 and $MgSO_4$). The spores obtained in Takashio broth were asexual conidia, but during parasitism, the organism produces more arthroconidia. The study of the enzyme activity of *T. rubrum* during arthroconidia formation (produced during parasitism) is not possible because of the nonavailability of techniques to induce arthroconidial formation *in vitro*. Therefore, the low levels of protease activity of *T. rubrum* during sporulation phase cannot be directly correlated with pathogenesis.

Nevertheless, it is really intriguing to know the reason for low protease production during sporulation in all the anthropophilic groups of dermatophytes when the geophilic and zoophilic organisms showed almost statistically comparable levels of protease production during both the phases of growth [26]. Is this moderation of enzyme activity during sporulation an adaptation of well-defined anthropophization?

12. Protease in *M. furfur* and pathogenesis

Enzyme secretion is regarded as one of the prominent virulence factors that are exhibited by many pathogens. Protease is an important virulence factor in several yeasts, including infections caused by *Candida* species in humans [27, 28] and keratinolytic proteases of *Candida albicans* is involved in the invasion and digestion of human stratum corneum *in vitro* [29]. Lipases produced by *Malassezia* are generally considered to be potential pathogenic factors. However, Coutinho and Paula [30] had reported that all the strains of *Malassezia pachydermatis* isolated from dogs showed protease activity. Protease released by *Malassezia* species was proposed as the mediator of itch at free nerve endings in the skin and a contributor to the prominent pruritus seen in affected dogs [31]. Members of the genus *Malassezia* are reported to have a role in inflammatory to mild scalp conditions such as seborrheic dermatitis and dandruff, besides being implicated in pityriasis versicolor.

Seborrheic dermatitis is characterized by inflammation and desquamation in areas that are rich in sebaceous glands, such as the scalp, face, and upper trunk. Dandruff is a major cosmetic concern with noninflammatory scaling conditions of the scalp [32, 33]. The importance of *Malassezia* organisms in these scalp conditions has been supported by studies demonstrating parallel decreases in the number of organisms and the severity of the diseases [34, 35]. *Malassezia* organisms produce lipases, which can alter sebum production in the host and can produce break-out products such as free fatty acids on the skin surface, which is responsible for the clinical conditions [36]. *M. pachydermatis* strains are known to produce proteases that are linked to its parasitic mode of life [37].

The protease activity of the isolates of *M. furfur* from different clinical conditions, such as pityriasis versicolor, dandruff, and seborrheic dermatitis, showed varied activity. The protease production is mild from isolates of pityriasis versicolor, high in dandruff, and very high in seborrheic dermatitis (**Table 3**).

It is interesting to note that the low protease activity of *M. furfur* isolates corresponds to the chronicity of pityriasis infection, which is in a similar line to that of *T. rubrum* isolates from chronic cases of dermatophytosis. Ranganathan et al. [24] reported a similar finding on the relationship between chronicity and the low protease profile of *T. rubrum* isolates. The protease activity is high in isolates of seborrheic dermatitis, which again corresponds to the high level of inflammation in the patients.

Clinical conditions	Enzyme activity (units)	
	Mean	SD
Seborrheic dermatitis	188.57	91.51
Pityriasis versicolor	42.61	15.46
Dandruff	140.36	62.60
F-value	37.075	
P-value	0.000	

Table 3.
Comparative enzyme activity in M. furfur isolates from different clinical conditions.

The role of protease in pathogenesis or severity of infection caused by *M. furfur* is not clearly known; however, studies of Gokulshankar [16] throw light on the possible role. However, in the earlier study conducted by Chen et al. [38], the culture extracts of *Malassezia* sp. with and without proteases failed to stimulate canine keratinocytes *in vitro.* Probably, the combined activity of lipases and proteases is responsible for the clinical condition caused by *M. furfur.*

13. Pigment production in *T. rubrum*

T. rubrum is a typical example of an anthropophilic dermatophyte that is globally prevalent. Several studies from different geographical locations have documented that *T. rubrum* is one among the predominant dermatophyte species, which is the most frequent cause of human dermatophyte infections. As early as 1982, [39] have reported the ability of this species to cause persistent infection, which is often found to be refractory to treatment.

The unique feature, which differentiates *T. rubrum* from other species of dermatophyte, is the cherry red pigment produced by the organism. It is a useful tool for the identification of this species in conventional diagnostic mycology. The question that remains unanswered is: what is the role of the pigments in pathogenesis? Rippon [3] has reported that *T. rubrum* var. *nigricans* cause a severe lesion in humans when compared to the usual variety of *T. rubrum*. However, the nature of the pigment produced by *T. rubrum* and the external factors that influence the pigment production in *T. rubrum* are not clearly understood. Interestingly, during pigment production, the enhanced sporulation of the fungus has been noted [5]. Further enhanced sporulation is seen during active parasitism [3].

Gokulshankar [16] found that the color and nature of the pigment released by *T. rubrum* during sporulation and vegetative phase were different. However, both the pigments were highly soluble in methanol:chloroform (1:1) solution. The single band of pigment released during the sporulation phase was similar to that of one of the bands of the two fractions of the pigment released during the vegetative phase when run on thin-layer chromatography (TLC) plate. Furthermore, these two bands showed fluorescence under UV light. However, earlier studies [40] indicate that bands produced by *T. rubrum* in the different phases have a different spectral pattern, suggesting that the chemical nature of the pigment released by the organism during the sporulation phase is totally different from the vegetative phase. However, a detailed study on the chemistry of the pigment may establish its probable role in pathogenesis.

Gokulshankar [16] also employed the susceptibility pattern of pigment-producing and non-pigment-producing isolates of *T. rubrum* against the antifungals, such as griseofulvin and miconazole, as a measure to correlate pigment production to pathogenesis. It is interesting to note that the pigment-producing variants are less susceptible when compared to the non-pigment-producing isolates. However, how these pigments interfere with the antifungals to promote resistance in *T. rubrum* isolates is not clearly known and warrants a detailed study.

14. Role of melanin in *C. neoformans*

One important characteristic of *C. neoformans* that differentiates its pathogenic isolates from the nonpathogenic isolates and other *Cryptococcus* species is its ability to form a brown to black pigment (melanin) on any medium that contains diphenolic compounds (such as cowitchseed/niger seed/bird seed or caffeic acid agar) [7, 41]. This pigment was first described by Staib [42]. The importance of melanin production in *C. neoformans* virulence was first demonstrated by several workers. Rhodes et al. [43] reported that naturally occurring *C. neoformans* mutants lacking melanin (Mel) were less virulent in the mice model than the strains that produce melanin. Other researchers further established this fact [44, 45].

C. neoformans melanogenesis is capable of conversion of dihydroxyphenols (DOPA to dopaquinone). This conversion is catalyzed by a phenoloxidase, which is present in *C. neoformans*, and this conversion is a rate-limited step because subsequent steps in the melanin pathway are spontaneous, such as (a) dopaquinone rearranging to dopachrome and (b) subsequent autoxidation to melanin [46]. However, *C. neoformans* does not possess the tyrosinase enzyme. The absence of tyrosinase makes *C. neoformans* incapable of endogenous production of DOPA [45]. Therefore, the organism has to be grown in a medium containing diphenolic compounds (such as bird seed agar) to produce melanin. In the environment, if *C. neoformans* isolates are able to acquire diphenolic compounds, it is possible for the organism to produce melanin with phenoloxidase. The human brain is usually rich in catecholamines (such as DOPA) and, therefore, becomes an ideal (or is it favorite?) target site for infection (cryptococcal meningitis) by *C. neoformans.* However, the deterrent factor is that *C. neoformans* cannot use catecholamines as sole the carbon source of living. Hence, it is to be understood that the brain is not a preferred "nutritional niche" for the growth of *C. neoformans* [47]; rather, it may be rightly called a "survival niche." Melanin production is, thus, a virulence factor in the pathogenesis providing a survival advantage in meningeal infections. *C. neoformans* is most likely able to use catecholamines in the brain to become melanized, thereby capable of protecting itself from oxidative damage.

Melanin-producing isolates have several advantages as they were resistant to damage by an *in vitro* epinephrine oxidative system [47] and were found to be protected from damage by hypochlorite and permanganate [48]. Thus, *C. neoformans* mutants lacking phenoloxidase enzyme are highly susceptible both in the natural habitat and in the host tissue when the environment is hostile (decreased chance of survival).

Wang and Casadevall [49] added to the knowledge by testing the survival of *C. neoformans* in the presence of reactive nitrogen intermediates, nitric oxide, and the epinephrine oxidative system. Wang and Casadevall [50, 51] experimentally proved the survival advantage by culturing *C. neoformans* cells in a medium containing L-DOPA to allow them to produce melanin. Melanized *Cryptococci* survived damage in the test systems, which was significantly better than nonmelanized cells of the same strain.

Furthermore, in the human host, melanin production makes *C. neoformans* less susceptible to amphotericin B than nonmelanized yeast cells, and this may contribute to the challenge in the management of cryptococcal infections in immunocompromised hosts [50, 51].

Gokulshankar [16] demonstrated that melanin-producing clinical variants are more resistant to antifungals, viz., flucytosine and amphotericin B, than the non-pigment-producing environmental isolates. The clinical isolates were basically from AIDS cases, and their ability to produce melanin in defined minimal media containing DOPA and in caffeic acid agar combined with less susceptibility to standard antifungals is of greater significance.

The co-inoculation studies of *C. neoformans* with *C. lunata* also gave interesting results [16]. The colony of *C. lunata* was found to overgrow and inhibit the colony of *C. neoformans*. However, this phenomenon was observed only when the environmental isolates of *C. neoformans* were co-inoculated with *C. lunata*. The clinical isolates of *C. neoformans* showed a pattern of co-dominance (mutual inhibition of colonies at a distance) when grown on SDA with *C. lunata*. This pattern was unique as the environmental isolates used in the study were nonpigment producers (mel-) and the clinical isolates were pigment producing (mel+). *C. lunata* also produces a black pigment (similar to melanin?). It could be that the pigment produced by *C. lunata* is the inhibiting factor for nonmelanized cells of *C. neoformans*, whereas the melanin-producing *C. neoformans* shows co-dominance with the *C. lunata* because there is a mutual inhibition among the organisms at a distance. This clearly suggests that melanin production in *C. neoformans* is a key factor to survive the competition of the other fungi/bacteria in its environmental niche. *C. neoformans* is usually found in its natural environment, viz., pigeon coups in the melanized state [52].

The feeding assay of *C. neoformans* by earthworms showed that both the non-pigment-producing environmental isolates got digested in the gut of all the four species of earthworms, while the recovery of the pigment-producing clinical isolates was possible from all four species of earthworms. It can be, therefore, presumed that the melanization of *C. neoformans* may help not only in the UV protection as reported by earlier workers but also in escaping the predation by soil organisms such as earthworms.

In summary, melanin production in *C. neoformans* may have multiple functions. It is not only essential for protecting this opportunistic pathogen from host defenses but also provides a survival advantage in the environment (**Figures 1** and **2**).

It makes sense if the clinical isolates of *C. neoformans* are virulent, but Casadevall and Perfect (1998) found that isolates from soil samples are virulent. The environmental isolates are found to have two important traits: capsule and melanin production. It stimulated the interest of several researchers who put forth the following questions: (i) why does a soil/environment dwelling organism, such as *C. neoformans*, need to possess virulence characteristics and (ii) how did this organism acquire the ability to cause infections in animals and humans when the passage through them (as intermediate host/vector) is not required for their replication or survival?

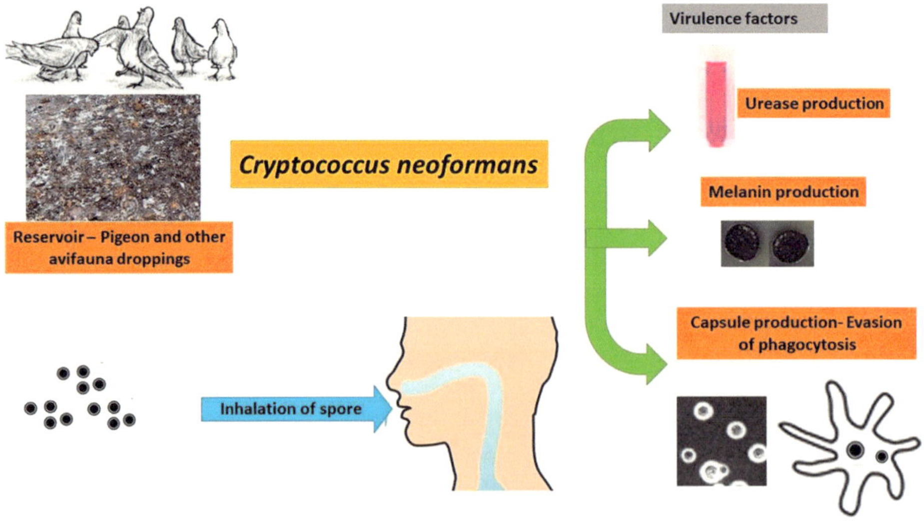

Figure 1.
Cryptococcus neoformans and its virulence factors.

DOI: http://dx.doi.org/10.5772/intechopen.105206

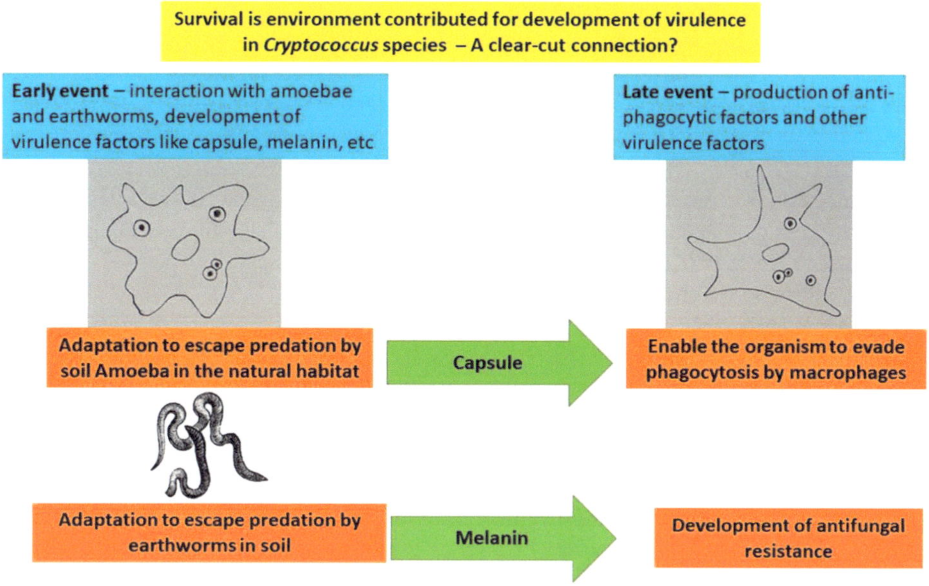

Figure 2.
Cryptococcus neoformans: Plausible factors that lead to the development and maintenance of virulence in the environment.

Bunting et al. [53] suggested that certain types of amoebae, *Acanthamobae polyphage*, can predate on *C. neoformans.* Steenbergen et al. [54] proposed that *C. neoformans* cells are phagocytosed by *A. castellani* and demonstrated the intracellular replication of yeast cells by the process of budding inside the phagosomes of the amoebae. They also did immunofluorescence microscopy and immunogold transmission electron microscopy to prove that the formation of polysaccharide-containing vesicles is associated with the intracellular growth of *C. neoformans* in amoebae. The phenomenon is similar to the one that is observed during the growth of *C. neoformans* in macrophages.

Melanin production, capsule synthesis, and phospholipase secretion were, therefore, required to escape the predation by amoebae. Therefore, the soil amoebae influence the survival traits of *C. neoformans*, which helps the organism for maintenance of the fungal virulence in the environment. Gokulshankar [16] demonstrated that the predation and digestion of nonmelanized cells are possible by four species of earthworms. Therefore, it is scientifically possible to consider the role of earthworms in maintaining of the virulence of *C. neoformans* in soil as well.

Further experiments of Rosas and Casadevall [55] confirmed that *in vitro* melanization makes *C. neoformans* less susceptible to hydrolytic enzymes. A feeding assay of C. *neoformans* with four different species of earthworms was carried out, and a similar kind of protection from the digestive enzymes of the earthworms could be the plausible reason for the recovery of only melanized cells of *C. neoformans* from the worm cast [16].

Melanin may also play a role in the protection of *C. neoformans* from the digestive enzymes released by the antagonistic microbes (soil fungi and bacteria) and provides a survival advantage during the constant and complex interactions of *C. neoformans* with other soil micro and macroflora.

15. Dimorphism and *H. capsulatum*

The ability of the fungus to have a morphologic transition from a geophilic (saprobe lifestyle) multicellular mold form to a parasitic (pathogenic/infective form) unicellular yeast form is called dimorphism. This phenomenon is governed by temperature in *H. capsulatum.* This MY shift (mold-to-yeast conversion) is an important virulence factor, and isolates that are incapable of this shift are avirulent [3].

This process can be replicated in the microbiology laboratory by just changing the incubation temperatures from room temperature 25°C (saprobic phase) to 37°C (parasitic phase), and the shift is usually reversible.

H. capsulatum is able to produce a defect in macrophages by shutting down the respiratory burst activity, which is key microbicidal activity to address the intracellular pathogens. Histoplasmosis, in general, considered the "fungal equivalent" (homolog) to the bacterial infection (tuberculosis) caused by *Mycobacterium tuberculosis.* Interestingly, both *H. capsulatum* and *M. tuberculosis* are capable of exploiting the immune cells of the host (macrophage) and using them as a vehicle for causing infections (acute or persistent pulmonary and its dissemination to the organ system [56].

Gokulshankar [16] wanted to find whether yeast form is more pathogenic than mold form. However, we have demonstrated experimentally that intracellular growth inside macrophages is not only possible for yeast form of *H. capsulatum* but also for the mold form. The yeast cells get converted to mold form (observed as formation of hyphae) in the macrophages at an incubation temperature of 25°C. This shift from yeast to mold form inside macrophages indicates that the mold form could also be equally infective. However, due to the constant body temperature of 37°C of the human host, which favors yeast growth, mold form is seldom encountered in the human tissues during infection. The infectivity of the mold form of *H. capsulatum* is further confirmed by infection assay in garden lizard (poikilothermic animal model), where experimental lesions are possible by injecting mold/yeast form and incubating the animal at both 25°C and 37°C. The saprophytic survival of the yeast form is not possible for *H. capsulatum.* The existence of the yeast form of *H. capsulatum* in

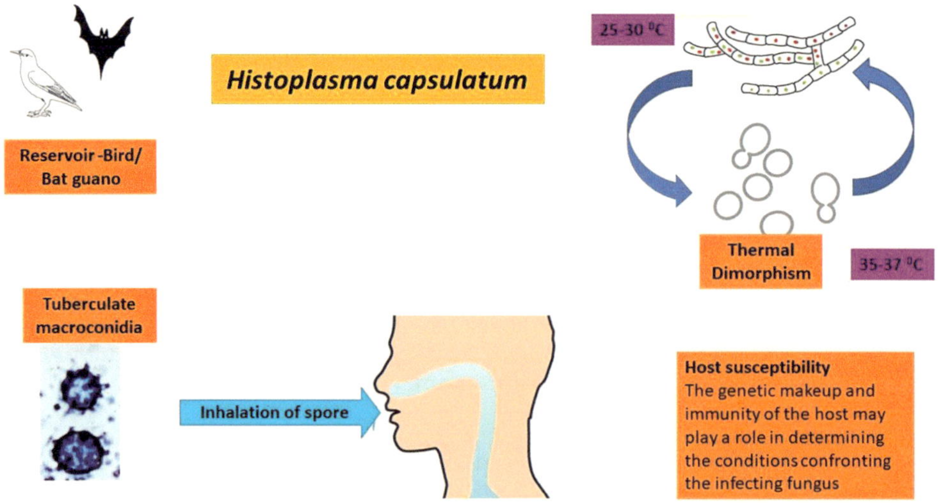

Figure 3.
Histoplasma capsulatum and its virulence factors.

the soil is challenged by predating organisms such as earthworms (may be also by soil amoebae as in the case of *C. neoformans*). The yeast cells of *H. capsulatum* get digested inside the gut of earthworms, and their recovery was not possible. The mold form of *H. capsulatum* survives predation by earthworms. This could be attributed to the formation of ornamented macroconidia (tuberculate) by the mold culture of *H. capsulatum*. Probably, in the course of evolution, *H. capsulatum* managed to adapt itself for intracellular growth (inside phagocytic cells) by developing intracellular yeast form, while a mold form is inevitable for existence as a saprophyte in soil. The compact yeast form may be more resistant to the enzymatic degradation in the intracellular state than a mold form. Eissenberg et al. [57] proposed that yeast cells of *C. neoformans* adapt the mechanism of increasing the pH of the phagolysosome to manage and survive in the otherwise extremely hostile environment is by increasing the pH of the phagolysosome. Thus, dimorphism gives the advantage to *H. capsulatum* for two modes of survival: parasitic (as yeast) and saprophytic (as mold) (**Figure 3**).

16. Conclusion

The ecological niche of different groups of dermatophytes varies from species to species. For example, in the genus *Microsporum*, *N. gypsea* is geophilic, while *M. canis* is zoophilic despite the fact that both of these organisms are basically keratinophilic in nature. For a long time, no clear-cut answer was previously given for how and why such a unique divergence in their habitat preference has emerged. Several studies have established the existence of homology at the genetic level between the geophilic

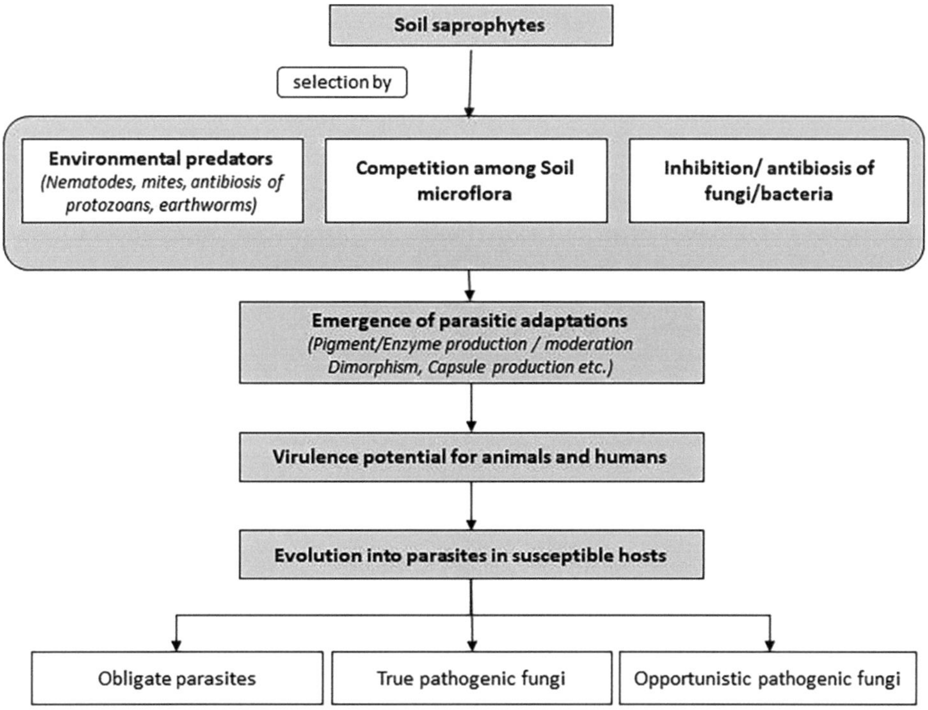

Figure 4.
Proposed probabilities of the evolution of saprophytic fungi into pathogenic fungi.

dermatophytes and the highly evolved "present-day" obligate parasitic dermatophytes. Mycologists strongly believe that these anthropophilic parasites might have existed in the soil before and gradually lost all these soil-inhabiting characteristics in their process of evolution as obligate parasites.

In the light of the findings of Gokulshankar et al, it is presumed that the inability of anthropophilic dermatophytes to escape the predation or manage to survive in the earthworm gut might have also contributed to the shrinkage of their prevalence in earthworm-rich soils, and therefore, these dermatophytes would have been forced to select a new line of adaptation. The ubiquitous prevalence of different species of earthworms in the majority of soil types all over the world is known, and this fact makes it possible to hypothesize that these once saprophytic dermatophytes would have the chance to pass through the gut of earthworms during their existence in soil. Probably, their inability to escape the predation (unable to survive successfully in the gut during this passage) could have also contributed to their elimination from the natural habitat. Other contributing factors could be the antidermatophytic activity of the predominant keratinophilic fungi in soil (such as *C. keratinophillum*). This inhibition coupled with antibiosis by other soil fungi (such as *Aspergillus* species) could also have played a role in the parasitic divergence of these dermatophytes. The role of other soil macroflora, such as mycophagous insects and mites, cannot be ruled out.

Similarly, the predation by earthworms (also by other nematodes and amoebae) may help in the maintenance of virulence in saprophytically existing pathogens such as *C. neoformans* and *H. capsulatum* (**Figure 4**).

Conflict of interest

None to declare.

The major part of this chapter is an extract from the PhD work of the first author.

Note

At the time of conduction of this experiment, *M. furfur* was commonly implicated with dandruff, but according to the new classification method of molecular biology, currently, *M. globosa* and *M. restricta* are both attributed to dandruff and other scalp conditions caused by these lipophilic yeasts.

Author details

Gokul Shankar Sabesan[1]*, Ranjit Singh Aja[2], Ranjith Mehenderkar[3] and Basanta Kumar Mohanty[4]

1 Faculty of Medicine, Department of Microbiology, Manipal University College Malaysia, Melaka, Malaysia

2 Department of Biotechnology, Prathyusha Engineering College Chennai, India

3 Faculty of Medicine, Deputy Dean- Preclinical, Quest International University Perak, Malaysia

4 Faculty of Medicine, Department of Pharmacology, Manipal University College Malaysia, Melaka, Malaysia

*Address all correspondence to: gokul.shankar@manipal.edu.my; gokkavi@gmail.com.

References

[1] GokulShankar S, Ranganathan S, Ranjith MS, Ranjithsingh AJA. Prevalence, serotypes and mating patterns of *Cryptococcus neoformans* in the pellets of different avifauna in Madras, India. Mycoses. 2004;**47**:310-314

[2] Gokulshankar S, Remya V, Ranjithsingh AJA, Ranjith MS. Does competition for existence pushed the evolution of the 'once' saprophytic fungi to parasitic life? Malaysian Journal of Microbiology. 2015;**11**(3):54-69

[3] Rippon JW. Medical Mycology, the Pathogenic Fungi and Pathogenic Actionmycetes. 3rd ed. Philadelphia: W.B. Saunders; 1988

[4] Weitzman I, Summerbell RC. The dermatophytes. Clinical Microbiology Reviews. 1995;**8**(2):240-259

[5] Ranganathan S. Characterization of Dermatophytes by Biotyping, Mating Experiments, DNA Typing and Protease Profile and the Possible Therapeutic Efficasy of *Azadirachta indica* in the Treatment of Tinea Infections. Ph.D thesis. Madras, India: University of Madras; 1996

[6] Tanaka S, Summerbell RC, Tsuboi R, Kaaman T, Sohnle G, Matsumoto T, et al. Advances in dermatophytes and dermatophytosis. Journal of Medical and Veterinary Mycology. 1992;**30** (Suppl. 1):29-39

[7] Kwon-Chung KJ. Cryptococcosis. In: Kwon-Chung KJ, Bennett JE, editors. Medical Mycology. Philadelphia: Lea & Febiger; 1992. pp. 397-446

[8] Armstrong PA, Jackson BR, Haselow D, Fields V, Ireland M, Austin C, et al. Multistate epidemiology of histoplasmosis, United States, 2011-2014. Emerging Infectious Diseases. 2018;**24**(3):425-431

[9] Lev S, Desmarini D, Li C, Chayakulkeeree M, Traven A, Sorrell TC, et al. Djordjevic phospholipase C of *Cryptococcus neoformans* regulates homeostasis and virulence by providing inositol trisphosphate as a substrate for Arg1 kinase. Infection and Immunity. 2013;**81**(4):1245-1255. DOI: 10.1128/IAI.01421-12

[10] Makimura M, Mochizuki T, Hasegawa A, Uchida K, Saito H, Yamaguchi H. Phylogenetic classification of *Trichophyton mentagrophytes* complex strains based on DNA sequences of nuclear ribosomal internal transcribed spacer 1 regions. Journal of Clinical Microbiology. 1998;**36**:2629-2633

[11] Makimura M, Tamura Y, Mochizuki T, et al. Phylogenetic classification and species identification of dermatophyte strains based on DNA sequences of nuclear ribosomal internal transcribed spacer 1 regions. Journal of Clinical Microbiology. 1999;**37**:920-924

[12] Summerbell RC, Haugland R, Li A, Gupta AK. Ribosomal RNA internal transcribed spacer 1 and 2 sequences of asexual, anthropophilic dermatophytes related to *Trichophyton rubrum*. Journal of Clinical Microbiology. 1999;**37**:4005-4011

[13] GokulShankar S, Ranjithsingh AJA, Ranjith MS, Ranganathan S, Palaniappan R. Role of *Chrysosporium keratinophillum* in the parasitic evolution of dermatophytes. Mycoses. 2005;**48**:1-5

[14] GokulShankar S, Ranjith MS, Ranganathan S, Selvakumar BN,

Aejaz M. Influence of *Chrysosporium* spp. in the prevalence of dermatophytes in soil. Indian Journal of Dermatology. 2001;**46**(3):142-145

[15] Deshmukh SK, Agarwal SC. Isolation of dermatophytes and other keratinophilic fungi from soils of Jammu, India. Mycoses. 2004;**46**:226-228

[16] Gokulshankar S. Parasitism in Certain Pathogenic Fungi – Evolutionary Aspects and Parasitic Adaptations. Ph.D thesis. Tirunelveli, India: Manonmanium Sundaranar University; 2007

[17] Shankar SG, Ranganathan S, Ranjith MS, Vijayalakshmi GS. Did earthworms contribute to the parasitic evolution of dermatophytes? Mycoses. 2002;**45**:399-401

[18] Steenbergen JN, Casadevall A. The origin and maintenance of virulence for the human pathogenic fungus *Cryptococcus neoformans*. Microbes and Infection. 2003;**5**:667-675

[19] Ogawa H, Nozawa Y, Rojanavanich V, et al. Fungal enzymes in the pathogenesis of fungal infections. Journal of Medical and Veterinary Mycology. 1992;**30**(1):189-196

[20] Ruchel R, Boning B, Jahn E, et al. Identification and partial charcarctyerization of two protenases from the cell envelope of *Candida albicans* blastospores. Zentralblatt Fur Bacteriologie Mikrobiologie and Hygiene, A. 1985;**260**:523-538

[21] Wretlind B, Wadstrom T. Purification and properties of a protease with elastase activity from *Pseudomonas aeruginosa*. Journal of General Microbiology. 1977;**103**:319-327

[22] Lu YC. A new method for the study of hair digestion by dermatophytes. Mycopathologia et mycologia applicata. 1962;**17**:225-235

[23] Minocha Y, Pasricha JS, Mohapatra LN, et al. Proteolytic activity of dermatophytes and its role in the pathogenesis of skin lesions. Sabouraudia. 1972;**18**:79-128

[24] Ranganathan S, Ranjith MS, GokulShankar S, Arun Mozhi Balajee S, Selvakumar BN, Aejaz M. Protease production in dermatophytes during sporulation and vegetative phase-its role in pathogenesis and mating type associated virulence. Indian Journal of Dermatology. 2000;**45**(4):174-181

[25] Fisher F, Cook NB. Fundamentals of Diagnostic Mycology. Philadelphia: WB saunders Company; 1998

[26] Gokulshankar S, Ranjitsingh AJA, Venkatesan G, Ranjith MS, Vijayalakshmi GS, Prabhamanju M, et al. Is moderation of protease production an adaptation of well-defined anthropization in dermatophytes? Indian Journal of Pathology and Microbiology. 2010;**53**(1):87-92

[27] Cassone A, De Bernardis F, Mondello F, et al. Evidence for a correlation between proteinase secretion and vulvovaginal candidiasis. Journal of Infectious Diseases. 1987;**156**:777-783

[28] Macdonald F, Odds FC. Virulence for mice of a proteinase- secreting strain of *Candida albicans* and a proteinase-deficient mutant. Journal of General Microbiology. 1983;**129**:431-438

[29] Negi M, Tsuboi R, Matsui T, Ogawa H. Isolation and characterization of proteinase from *Candida albicans*: Substrate specificity. Journal of Investigative Dermatology. 1984;**83**:32-36

[30] Coutinho SD, Paula CR. Proteinase, phospholipase, hyaluronidase and

chondroitin-sulphatase production by *Malassezia pachydermatis*. Medical Mycology. 2000;**38**:73-76

[31] Mason KV, Evans AG. Dermatitis associated with *Malassezia pachydermatis* in eleven dogs. Journal of the American Animal Hospital Association. 1991;**27**:13-20

[32] Chen T, Hill PB. The biology of *Malassezia* organisms and their ability to induce immune responses and skin disease. Veterinary Dermatology. 2005;**16**:4-26

[33] Hay RJ, Graham-Brown RA. Dandruff and seborrhoeic dermatitis: Causes and management. Clinical and Experimental Dermatology. 1997;**22**:3-6

[34] Heng MC, Henderson CL, Barker DC, et al. Correlation of *Pityrosporum ovale* density with clinical severity of seborrhoeic dermatitis as assessed by a simplified technique. Journal of the American Academy of Dermatology. 1990;**23**:82-86

[35] Pierard-Franchimont C, Arrese JE, Durupt G, et al. Correlation between *Malassezia* spp. load and dandruff severity. Journal of de Mycologie Medicale. 1998;**8**:83-86

[36] Mason IS, Mason KV, Lloyd DH. A review of the biology of canine skin with respect to the commensals *Staphylococcus intermedius*, *Demodex canis* and *Malassezia. Pachydermatis*. Veterinary Dermatology. 1996;**7**:119-132

[37] Nicklas D, Buse M. Proteolyse of *Pityrosporum pachydermatis* strains. Mykosen. 1982;**25**:633-637

[38] Chen T, Halliwell REW, Hill PB. Failure of extracts from *Malassezia pachydermatis* to stimulate canine keratinocyte proliferation *in vitro*. Veterinary Dermatology. 2002;**13**:323-329

[39] Hay RJ, Shennan G. Chronic dermatophyte infection II. Antibody and cell mediated response. The British Journal of Dermatology. 1982;**106**:191-198

[40] Arunmozhi Balajee S. Studies on the Prevalence and Etiology of Dermatophytosis in Diabetics, Cancer and HIV/AIDS Patients, Carriage Rate in ABO Blood Groups and Characterization of Certain Dermatophytes. Ph.D Thesis. Madras India: University of Madras; 1998

[41] Williamson PR. Laccase and melanin in the pathogenesis of *Cryptococcus neoformans*. Frontiers in Bioscience. 1997;**2**:e99-e107

[42] Staib F. *Cryptococcus neoformans* and *Guizotia abyssinica*. Zeitschrift fur Hygiene. 1962;**148**:466-475

[43] Rhodes JC, Polacheck I, Kwon-Chung KJ. Phenoloxidase activity and virulence in isogenic strains of *Cryptococcus neoformans*. Infection and Immunity. 1982;**36**:1175-1184

[44] Salas SD, Bennett JE, Kwon-Chung KJ, Perfect JR, Williamson PR. Effect of the laccase gene, CNLACI, on virulence of *Cryptococcus neoformans*. The Journal of Experimental Medicine. 1996;**184**:377-386

[45] Torres-Guerrero H, Edman JC. Melanin deficient mutants of Cryptococcus neoformans. Journal of Medical and Veterinary Mycology. 1994;**32**:303-313

[46] Polacheck I, Kwon-Chung KJ. Melanogenesis in *Cryptococcus neoformans*. Journal of General Microbiology. 1988;**134**:1037-1041

[47] Polacheck I, Platt Y, Aronovitch J. Catecholamines and virulence of *Cryptococcus neoformans*. Infection and Immunity. 1990;**58**:2919-2922

[48] Jacobson ES, Tinnell SB. Antioxidant function of fungal melanin. Journal of Bacteriology. 1993;**175**:7102-7104

[49] Wang Y, Casadevall A. Susceptibility of melanized and nonmelanized *Cryptococcus neoformans* to nitrogen and oxygen-derived oxidants. Infection and Immunity. 1994c;**62**:3004-3007

[50] Wang Y, Casadevall A. Decreased susceptibility of melanized *Cryptococcus neoformans* to UV light. Applied and Environmental Microbiology. 1994a;**60**(10):3864-3866

[51] Wang Y, Casadevall A. Growth of *Cryptococcus neoformans* in presence of L-dopa decreases its susceptibility to amphotericin B. Antimicrobial Agents and Chemotherapy. 1994b;**38**:2648-2650

[52] Nosanchuk JD, Rudolph J, Rosas AL, Casadevell A. Evidence that *Cryptococcus neoformans* is melanized in pigeon excreta: Implications for pathogenesis. Infection and Immunity. 1999;**67**:5477-5479

[53] Bunting LA, Neilson JB, Bulmer GS. *Cryptococcus neoformans*: Gastronomic delight of a soil amoeba. Sabouraudia. 1979;**17**:225-232

[54] Steenbergen JN, Shuman HA, Casadevall A. *Cryptococcus neoformans* interactions with amoebae suggest an explanation for its virulence and intracellular pathogenic strategy in macrophages. Proceedings of National Academic Science USA. 2001;**98**:15245-15250

[55] Rosas AL, Casadecall A. Melanization decreases the susceptibility of *Cryptococcus neoformans* to enzymatic degradation. Mycopathologia. 2001;**151**:53-56

[56] Woods JP. *Histoplasma capsulatum* molecular genetics, pathogenesis, and responsiveness to its environment. Fungal Genetics and Biology. 2002;**35**(2):81-97

[57] Eissenberg LG, Goldman WE, Schlesinger PH. *Histoplasma capsulatum* modulates the acidification of phagolysosomes. The Journal of Experimental Medicine. 1993;**177**:1605-1611

Section 3

Parasitic Infectious Diseases

Chapter 5

Biology and Epidemiology of Malaria Recurrence: Implication for Control and Elimination

Aklilu Alemayehu

Abstract

Malaria recurrence not only increases its clinical episodes, but also sustains transmission. It significantly contributes to a high burden of malaria and impedes elimination. Malaria recurrence can be due to reinfection, relapse, or recrudescence. Based on the type of recurrence, parasites exhibit similar or dissimilar genotypes compared to the genotype involved in initial infection. This review aimed at showing a comprehensive overview of malaria recurrence. Molecular techniques, such as real-time polymerase chain reaction (PCR), nested PCR, multiplex PCR, and sequencing, help to characterize malaria recurrence. However, these tools are hardly accessible in malaria-endemic areas and are unable to detect liver hypnozoites. Moreover, PCR is unable to adequately differentiate between relapse and reinfection of *P. vivax*. Recurrent malaria, particularly relapse, accounts for major portion of malaria prevalence. Through renewed parasitemia, recurrence remained as a daunting public health problem. More works remain to overcome the challenges of recurrence in efforts to control and eliminate malaria. Limited understanding of malaria recurrence impedes the development of robust tools and strategies for effective mitigation. Continued biological and epidemiological studies help unravel the persistent complexities of malaria recurrence and develop ideal tool to fight malaria.

Keywords: *plasmodium*, recurrence, reinfection, recrudescence, relapse, malaria elimination

1. Introduction

Recurrence of malaria is the return of malaria symptoms after varying lengths of symptom-free duration [1]. It often involves the reappearance of asexual stages of *Plasmodium* parasite in the peripheral circulation of a person, who was previously infected [1–3]. The reappearing parasite can be either similar or different to the genotype and/or species of the parasite responsible for primary infection [1, 2, 4]. Reemergence of asexual parasitemia can be due to persistence of the asexual parasite despite treatment; release from liver schizogony of reactivated hypnozoite; or from a novel infection [1].

Relapse and recrudescence are forms of recurrent malaria involving renewed parasitemia following hypnozoite reactivation and unsuccessful treatment, respectively. Reinfection involves the reappearance of malaria ensuing from the inoculation of sporozoites from an infected mosquito bite. Generally, depending on its source, malaria recurrence is classified into three types: relapse, recrudescence, and reinfection [1, 2]. The source of recurrence can be assessed by combining clinical findings with microscopy, genotyping, and measuring drug absorption [5].

2. Biology of malaria recurrence

2.1 Reinfection

Reinfection is renewed clinical illness or peripheral blood parasitemia due to a new infection with *plasmodium* parasite [6]. It appears after recovery from the primary infection, but usually involves different genotypes of the parasite [1, 5]. Malaria reinfection results from the injection of new sporozoites. It is critical to identify reinfection from other types of malaria recurrence for public health decision-making [5].

Markers currently employed to distinguish reinfection from other types of malaria recurrence include merozoite surface proteins (MSP1 and MSP2) and the gene of the glutamate rich protein (GLURP) [5, 7]. In reinfection, the reappearing parasite should not always exhibit a different genotype from the organism found at initial infection [1, 2]. However, all alleles of the posttreatment appearing parasite should be distinct from those identified in the pretreatment sample tested for one or more loci. This means it is possible to declare reinfection based on a single marker exhibiting disparity on all of its alleles between pretreatment and posttreatment samples [5, 7].

Reinfection is often associated with *P. falciparum* in endemic settings [8]. However, emerging reports show the possibility of reinfection with other species of *Plasmodium* [8, 9]. Likewise, Lau *et al.*, reported reinfection with a nonhomologous strain of *Plasmodium knowlesi* from Malaysia [10]. In the case of *Plasmodium vivax*, reinfection could be disregarded if the patient relocates to settings with no malaria transmission [9]. Particular attention is vital to characterize involved species and the corresponding management [8]. Besides, reinfection further exacerbates transmission dynamics with its potential to activate hypnozoite; introduce new strains and/or species to result in heterologous relapse, and provide a chance for immune evasion. Generally, malaria recurrence increases efficiency, chance, and longevity of malaria transmission in so doing it threatens the productivity of interventions [11].

Reinfection can play a remarkable role in sustaining both the clinical and epidemiological impact of malaria. Reinfection with *P. vivax* entails relapse from itself and/or from the latent infection [9]. Similarly, reinfection with *P. falciparum* triggers relapse, thereby complicating the disease and the subsequent transmission potential [12]. In areas with high transmission of malaria, slowly eliminated antimalarial drugs are used to clear parasitemia and reduce the risk of subsequent reinfection [13]. Appropriate case management can potentially reduce parasite transmission [14]. Frequent reinfections can arise from the poor yield of interventions. Therefore, reinfection is a good marker for the effectiveness of preventive activities, such as vector control [9, 14, 15].

2.2 Relapse

Malaria relapse is hypnozoite-mediated reemergence of malaria symptoms following a successful clearance of bloodstream parasitemia. It is characterized by the recurrence of asexual parasitemia ascending from hypnozoite stages of past infection [1–3, 16]. The dormant hypnozoites persist in the liver and mature to form hepatic schizonts. These hepatic schizonts rupture and release merozoites into the peripheral circulation with an interval commonly ranging from 3 weeks to 1 year [1, 2, 17, 18]. Relapse is common in *P. vivax* and *Plasmodium ovale* infections [2, 16, 19].

Liver hypnozoites can be formed either at initial infection from the newly inoculated *Plasmodium* or during the existing infection from the erythrocytic *Plasmodium*. In areas where *P. falciparum* and *P. vivax* are co-endemic, the newly inoculated sporozoites of *P. vivax* sometimes directly go to the dormant stage in the liver as a strategy to avoid the potential damage that can result from the competition with *P. falciparum* in the bloodstream [20]. Reactivation of dormant hypnozoite occurs in response to the creation of favorable conditions due to various factors, such as a change in host immunity or inoculation of new *Plasmodium* [4, 12].

For a long time, relapse is considered as the hypnozoite-mediated reappearance of clinical malaria [16]. However, recent developments suggest the possibility of relapse from the reappearance of erythrocytic plasmodial stages from bone marrow and spleen. According to studies on nonhuman primates and humans, bone marrow is a key tissue reservoir of *P. vivax* schizonts [21–23]. Apart from a hypnozoite origin, another noncirculating source bringing about homologous parasitemia results in relapse-like *P. vivax* recurrences, which would better be regarded as recrudescence than relapse [6]. This concept raises the question of differentiating the parasite population arising from hypnozoite and non-hypnozoite-driven recurrences [22].

Recurrence from noncirculating and non-hypnozoite sources, adds to the longstanding complexities of malaria biology and epidemiology, particularly vivax malaria [6, 16, 19, 21, 23]. Peripheral parasitemia is a poor indicator of parasite biomass in a patient [6, 22, 23]. Therefore, assessing the involvement of the hematologic niche in malaria recurrence is gaining attention from the scientific community to improve the understanding of the pathogenesis of recurrence and reinforce the fight against malaria [3, 21–23].

Recurrences due to *P. vivax* can be homologous or heterologous, either of which can be reinfection, recrudescence, or relapse [4, 6, 22, 24]. Besides, different populations of hypnozoites derived from repeated inoculations can be found in the peripheral blood of a person [17]. This introduces difficulty in discerning the type of recurrence in *P. vivax* [4]. However, it is possible to consider most homologous recurrences as relapse provided recrudescence can be excluded in areas with high genetic diversity of *P. vivax* [4, 20]. Yet, relapse rates might be underrated since they can sometimes contribute to heterozygous recurrence due to polyclonal inoculum by a mosquito [4, 6, 17, 22].

The relapse of *P. vivax* usually ranges from weeks to a year [17, 20]. However, according to controlled human malaria infection, the frequency and number of relapses differ with host immunity and geographical location. In tropical areas, the risk of relapse is high with short intervals (less than a month); whereas temperate and subtropical areas are characterized by a lower risk of relapse recurring after a long latency (8–12 months) [17, 25]. Consistent with this, patients in regions of short relapse periodicity had a greater rate of *P. vivax* parasitemia than those in regions of long relapse periodicity (HR = 8.61 95% CI: 2.34–31.65; P = 0.001) [17]. In addition to places, the severity of relapse illness shortens the periodicity by activating more hypnozoites in the liver [20]. Conceivably, a modeling result shows a shorter latent period of hypnozoites increases *P. vivax* recurrence further reinforcing the problem (**Figure 1**) [26, 27].

2.3 Recrudescence

Recrudescence of malaria is the return of malaria symptoms after symptom-free periods. It is caused by parasites surviving in peripheral circulation despite treatment [1]. Recrudescence is characterized by the reappearance of genetically similar asexual stage parasites to the initial infection, usually due to incomplete therapy. In recrudescence, at least one allele at each locus is common to both paired samples collected at primary infection and recurrence [5, 16]. Recrudescence often results from incomplete clearance of asexual parasites by antimalarial drugs. It is common in infections with *P. malariae* and *P. falciparum* [1, 2].

Recrudescence associated with failure to prevent or cure malaria does not necessarily mean drug resistance. It can also be a temporary drug-associated quiescence, whereby ring stages of *P. falciparum* parasite in the RBCs become temporarily dormant ensuing exposure to artemisinin derivatives, such as dihydroartemisinin [28]. Based on this phenomenon, it is conceivable that early homologous recurrence of *P. vivax* might be misclassified as relapses while being recrudescence resulting from temporary drug-induced dormancy. In the absence of PQ therapy, the use of whole-genome analysis might help resolve such uncertainty [24]. Recrudescence should be properly characterized as it carries a considerable public health challenge (**Table 1**) [29].

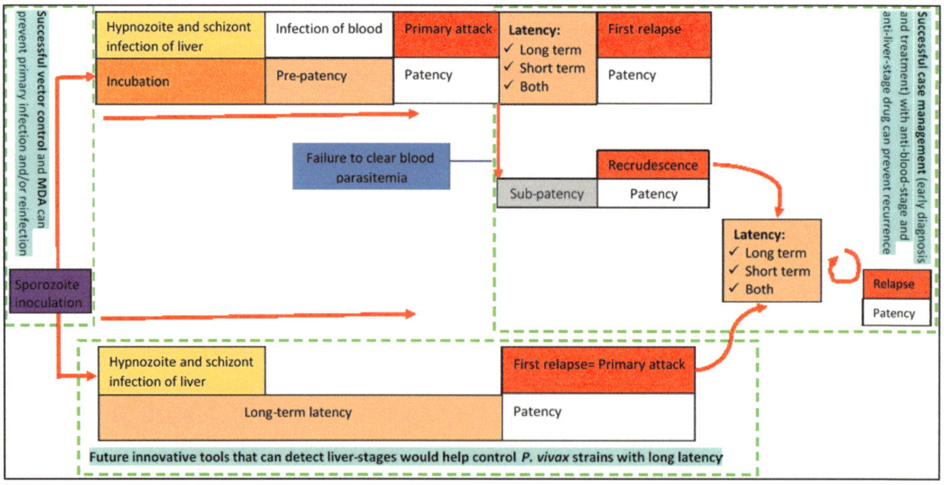

Figure 1.
Pathogenesis of infection, and recurrence with P. vivax. Hypnozoite and schizont infection of liver occur following inoculation of sporozoites. However, after the inoculation, the parasite may develop and multiply to cause blood infection (upper row) or may enter into long-term latency (lower row). Furthermore, a portion of the hypnozoites remains in the liver to continue to relapse periodically. Suggested intervention strategies at specific weak spots are indicated (green shades inside Brocken-lined boxes). MDA: Mass drug administration.

S. No	Feature	Relapse	Reinfection	Recrudescence	References
1	Genotype similarity to primary infection	Yes/No	No	Yes	[4, 5]
2	Periodicity	Weeks to years	Depends (multifactorial)	Days to weeks (Usually 3–4 weeks)	[9, 17]
3	Origin	Liver-hypnozoite	Sporozoites	Merozoites	[5, 6, 9]
4	Mechanism	Reactivation of liver-hypnozoite	Inoculation of sporozoites by bite from infected mosquito	Persistence of asexual parasitemia after treatment due to treatment failure	[3–6]
5	Need for mosquito bite	No	Yes	No	[5, 6]
6	Commonly involved species	*P. vivax* and *P. ovale*	*P. falciparum*	*P. falciparum* and *P. malariae*	[5, 6]

Table 1.
Comparison of different types of recurrence in malaria.

3. Management of malaria recurrence

3.1 Diagnosis of malaria recurrence

Proper laboratory diagnosis forms the foundation for achieving malaria control and elimination. Accurate, reliable, and timely results are essential to managing initial and recurrent episodes of malaria [30, 31]. The effectiveness of malaria intervention is a function of the right diagnosis at the right time and the right treatment. Treatment without laboratory confirmation may result in overtreatment with antimalarials that may facilitate the development of drug resistance and waste resources [8, 32]. Malaria case management solely based on a clinical diagnosis not only reduces the effectiveness of treatment outcomes but also worsens the clinical and epidemiological burden of malaria by paving the way for recurrence and transmission [8].

Malaria microscopy, so far, has been the mainstay to detect and identify *Plasmodium* parasites. However, this method suffers from deficiency to detect very low density of parasites and difficulty to identify recurrences [33]. Molecular diagnosis provides optimum sensitivity and specificity to characterize malaria recurrence. Distinguishing recrudescence from reinfection is important to monitor the effectiveness of the therapeutic intervention. Molecular tests, such as PCR, employ genotyping target genes of the *Plasmodium* for diagnosis of malaria recurrence [14, 32].

Genotyping *Plasmodium* parasites is fundamental to comprehending parasite biology; clinical management and innovation of tools to mitigate disease. *Plasmodium* parasites vary by pathogenesis; susceptibility to drugs; recurrence pattern; and transmissibility by mosquito species. Genotyping these parasites help to describe the current population, understand the relationship among various populations, and characterize clinical and epidemiological features [34]. The polymerase chain reaction is a powerful tool to detect and identify *Plasmodium* parasites with high sensitivity and high specificity, respectively [35]. Generally, genotyping stands at the forefront of malaria elimination [5, 33, 35].

Recent advances in molecular techniques have improved the detection and identification of malaria parasites [14, 34]. Unlike microscopy and rapid diagnostic tests (RDTs), molecular techniques involving PCR help to identify and characterize recurrences [30]. They are essential partners in the control and elimination of malaria, as they both help detect and prevent recurrence through increased sensitivity and specificity [34]. They help detection of sub-microscopic, asymptomatic, mixed, and multiclonal infections in addition to suggesting drug resistance possibility [36]. Hence, molecular techniques substantially improved case management by revealing these contributors to recurrence in various ways [30, 32].

Generally, although molecular tests ominously revolutionized the interventions against malaria, some works remain to further improve their yield in the fight against malaria. There is no reliable laboratory test to diagnose liver-stage hypnozoites of *P. vivax* [37]. Besides, in the case of *P. vivax*, it is difficult to differentiate between relapse, recrudescence, and reinfection, as they might involve parasites with similar or different genotypes to the parasite found in an initial infection. Due to their high cost and technical complexity, molecular tests are not readily available in developing countries with a high burden of malaria [5, 38].

3.1.1 Nested polymerase chain reaction

Nested PCR is a type of PCR that involves two sets of primers used in two sequential runs of PCR. It is a technique, whereby the first PCR generates a mix of all *Plasmodium* species DNA products, which can be used in the second PCR run with primers internal (nested) to the first pair of primers. The first amplification, nest 1, allows detection of the *Plasmodium* genus-specific genes. Products of samples tested positive will then be subjected to a further four nested reactions (for four species) to determine the species compositions [35]. The purpose of the second run is to amplify a secondary target (species-specific sequence) within the first run product. It is an ideal technique for increasing the sensitivity and specificity of PCR [5, 33, 35].

The nPCR assay genotypes malaria parasites by targeting marker genes for 18S rRNA, merozoite surface proteins (MSP1 and MSP2), and gene of the glutamate rich protein (GLURP). Detection of amplicons from nPCR is usually done by agarose gel electrophoresis. Besides, these markers help to discriminate recrudescence from reinfection [35]. These markers possess varying power to discriminate between *Plasmodium* species. Accordingly, while MSP2 and GLURP have similar power, MSP1 has lower discriminatory power than these two markers. Despite the vulnerability of GLURP to "artifact bands," and the varying performance of different markers across different geographical places, the general discriminatory power is constant [5].

Despite its remarkable benefits, nPCR is susceptible to contamination due to its extreme sensitivity and involvement in sample manipulation. Contamination originates from human errors due to the transfer of parasite material between samples or between samples and PCR reagents. The other type of contamination, which is more serious, occurs when PCR product from either of the two runs is exposed to samples, reagents, or equipment. Furthermore, the use of two separate reactions makes nPCR costly (**Figure 2**) [35].

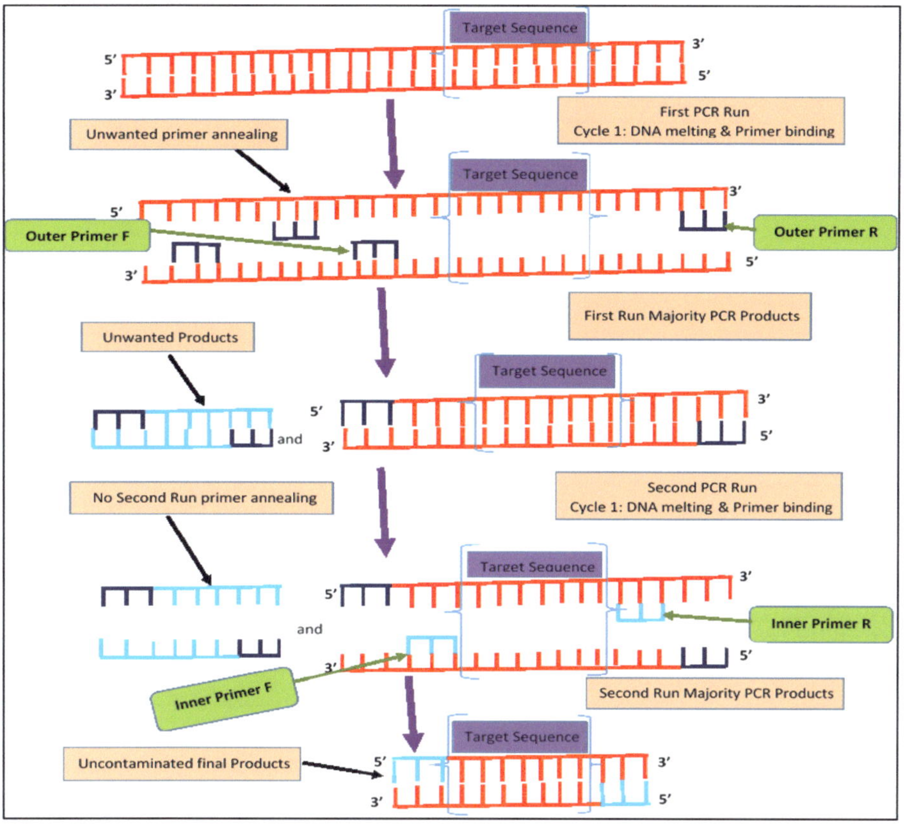

Figure 2.
Schematic diagram of nested PCR. The nPCR involves two-stage amplification of the target DNA of malaria parasites by using two sets of primers that target species- and genus-level markers of the plasmodium. The external primer targets genus-level-marker: 18S rRNA, whereas the internal primer targets species-level-marker: MSP1, MSP2, and GLURP. The first run may produce unwanted products. A portion of amplicons from the first run is used as a template in each of four separate PCR reactions to produce uncontaminated final products.

3.1.2 Real-time polymerase chain reaction

Real-time polymerase chain reaction (PCR) is usually referred to as quantitative PCR (qPCR) since it involves detection, identification, and quantification of target DNA data as it occurs. It is characterized by continuous monitoring of amplicons production from the parasite DNA by using fluorescent-labeled reporters, including DNA intercalating dyes, such as SYBR green, and sequence-specific probes [39]. Real-time PCR targets polymorphic regions of MSP1, MSP2, and GLURP and are present simultaneously or singly on the *Plasmodium* parasite [40].

Real-time PCR can play an important role in characterizing malaria recurrence through simultaneous detection and quantification of the *Plasmodium* parasite. It allows multiplexing that will provide a critical framework for the identification of parasites involved in reinfection, recrudescence, and relapse. Besides, as well as can help detect genes responsible for resistance to antimalarial drugs, thereby helping the chance of malaria recurrence and transmission [41–43]. Moreover, due to its good sensitivity and specificity, real-time qPCR can be useful in both epidemiological and clinical studies as well as early detection of cases that might entail recurrence (**Figure 3**) [44].

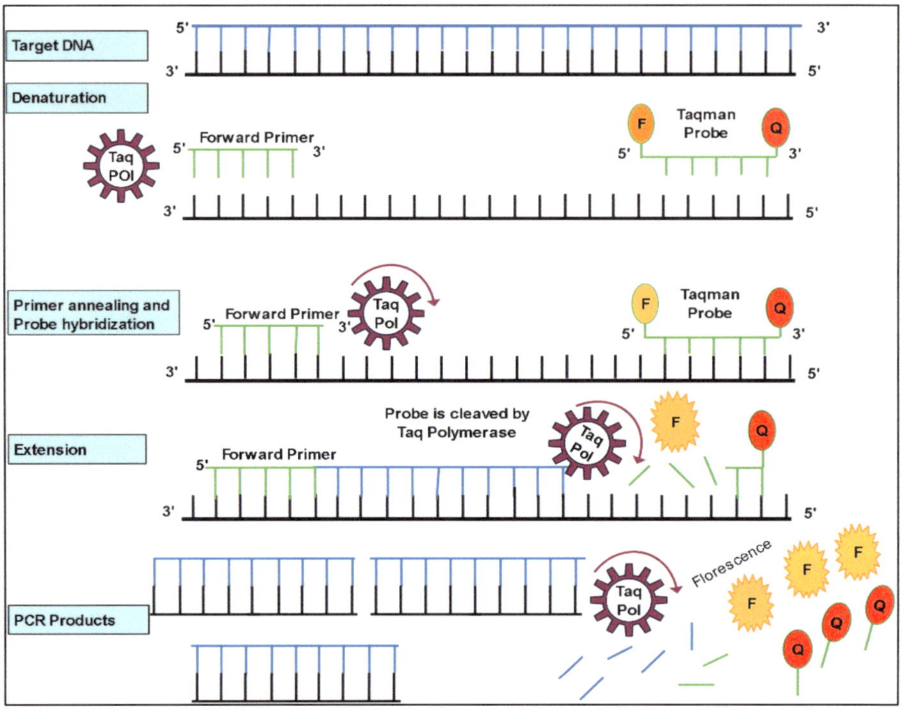

Figure 3.
Graphical presentation of real-time PCR principle (TaqMan system). Real-time PCR involves a probe that is labeled at the five prime ends with a fluorescent reporter dye (F) and at the three prime ends with a quencher dye (Q). In intact probes, the fluorescence of the reporter is quenched by the close presence of a quencher. Then, probes and the complementary DNA strand are hybridized and reporter fluorescence is still quenched. During extension step of the PCR, the probe is degraded by the Taq polymerase and the fluorescent reporter is released resulting in florescence emission, which is essential information to detect and quantify the target sequence. PCR: Polymerase chain reaction, Taq pol: Taq polymerase, Q: Quencher, and F: Fluorophore [42].

3.1.3 Multiplex polymerase chain reaction

Multiplex PCR is a molecular technique characterized by simultaneous detection of several targets within a single reaction by using diverse pairs of primers specifically designed for each target [41]. In context of malaria, specie-specific primers labeled with different fluorescent dyes targeting MSP and GLURP markers are contained in the master-mix used to detect five species of *Plasmodium* by a single run [40]. The recently developed multiplex malaria sample ready PCR showed a hopeful result in Sierra Leone by demonstrating twice and four times higher sensitivity compared to malaria RDT and microscopy, respectively [45].

Multiplex PCR provides more information with fewer samples in a reasonably short time. It allows the detection of multiple species of *Plasmodium* from a single sample with a single run, thereby contributing to characterizing types of recurrence for proper case management and research purpose. In general, multiplexing is an excellent cost-saving strategy, with a particular implication in resource-limited settings [40]. However, multiplex PCR suffers from process complexity, poor universality, and variability in efficiency for different templates. Furthermore, multiplex PCR showed relatively lower sensitivity than nPCR for *Plasmodium* species due to the competition between different amplicons for limited supplies found in the reaction well (**Figure 4**) [40, 47].

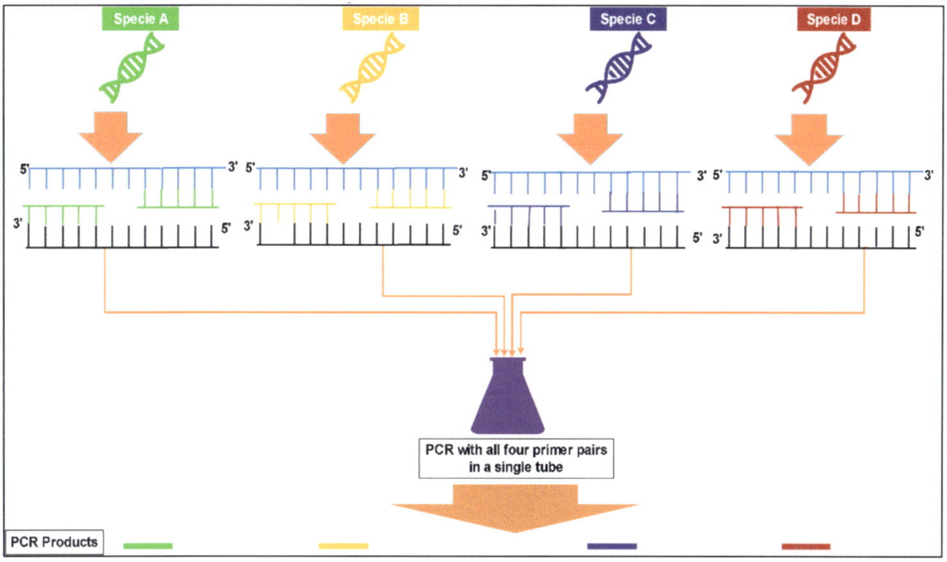

Figure 4.
Diagram showing the multiplex PCR approach [46]. Multiplex PCR is a type of PCR in which multiple target DNA are simultaneously amplified in a single reaction tube. It involves the use of specific primers that can specifically combine with their corresponding DNA target contained in a master-mix, and hence allow amplification of more than one DNA fragment from a single and/or many samples.

3.1.4 Sequencing

Sequencing is the process of determining the order of nucleotides in a piece of DNA. It can be done in a small targeted genomic region or entire genome of an organism, including *Plasmodium* parasite [48]. A single-cell level sequencing *Plasmodium* parasites to explore parasite relatedness in Malawi proved the possibility of emergence of a new strain within an individual from super-infection with *P. falciparum* due to repeated reinfection. This study also reported unexpectedly frequent co-transmission of related parasites in intense transmission settings in the country, thereby intensifying possibility of recurrence and transmission [49].

Whole genome sequencing of *P. vivax* isolates from Ethiopia revealed frequent sequence and structural polymorphisms in erythrocyte binding genes that code for Duffy antigen/chemokine receptors [50]. The currently emerging data suggest that MSP involved in RBC adhesion is rapidly evolving [50, 51]. This signals for expanding pattern of *P. vivax* in areas previously considered not affecting Duffy-negative individuals [50]. Moreover, sequencing data can help characterize recurrence, particularly strains involved in relapse, which is inevitable since the parasite continues to infect both Duffy-negative and positive people [50, 51].

Amplicon sequencing involves sequencing a particular DNA segment of a parasite we are interested in. It helps to identify a single nucleotide polymorphism in the *Plasmodium* parasite [52]. Amplicon sequencing helps to characterize the genetic diversity of *Plasmodium* parasites by showing the number of alleles in a population in time and space. It serves as an ideal tool for characterizing the spatiotemporal flow of *Plasmodium* infection and geographical tracking of transmission patterns, including new and recurrence [52]. It is also an important tool to assess drug resistance genes, particularly by detecting the kelch 13 (K13) propeller gene of *P. falciparum,* thereby allowing recrudescence characterization [53, 54]. Furthermore, next-generation sequencing enables determining the transmission dynamics of *Plasmodium* species [55]. Nevertheless, these parasite sequencing methods are costly and are not sufficiently standardized for extensive use in field and clinical settings, particularly in malaria-endemic settings (**Figure 5**) [52, 55].

3.2 Treatment and/or prevention of malaria recurrence

Primaquine is the only drug widely applied to prevent relapse by clearing liver hypnozoites [27]. Recently shreds of evidence are emerging on the possibility of preventing malaria relapse with a single dose tafenoquine (TQ) treatment [56]. Universal radical cure with ACT and PQ/TQ is hoped to reduce parasitemia by leveraging the high risk of *P. vivax* parasitemia following *P. falciparum* infection in co-endemic settings [57]. This strategy produced a remarkable reward within one year by bringing about a 90% reduction in parasitemia of *P. vivax* among a cohort of children in Papua New Guinea [17, 58].

Preventing recurrent parasitemia reduces morbidity and mortality directly associated with malaria and indirectly with other secondary diseases [59]. Besides, a comprehensive treatment policy for malaria provides considerable benefits at an individual, public health, and operational level in settings, where *P. falciparum* and *P. vivax* are co-endemic. For prevention of recurrence, particularly relapse of *P. vivax*, establishing strong adherence to a full dose of PQ as a radical cure can strengthen control and elimination efforts [37]. Individuals carrying a high load of hypnozoites are more likely to relapse and therefore be targeted for treatment with PQ [60].

Improved case management is pivotal to prevention and control of malaria recurrence, particularly recrudescence. Use of highly sensitive molecular tools, such as PCR, help to detect submicroscopic parasitemia, and hence treatment [8, 31]. On the other hand, strengthening vector control strategies is important to prevent reinfection by protecting from infectious mosquito bites [8].

Hypnozoiticidal therapy against latency is used to prevent relapses from *P. vivax* and *P. ovale* [7]. The G-6-PD status of patients should guide the administration of PQ to prevent relapse. To prevent relapse, treat *P. vivax* or *P. ovale* malaria in children and adults with a 14-day course (0.25–0.5 mg/kg/BW/day) of PQ in all transmission settings. Nevertheless, this recommendation excludes pregnant women, infants aged below 6 months, women breastfeeding infants aged below 6 months, women breastfeeding older infants with unknown G-6-PD status, and people with G-6-PD deficiency. In people with G-6-PD deficiency, with close medical supervision for the risk of PQ-provoked hemolysis, consider preventing relapse by giving PQ base at 0.75 mg/kg/BW/week for 8 weeks. If the G-6-PD status is unknown and G-6-PD testing is not available, a decision to prescribe PQ must be based on risks and benefits [37, 61].

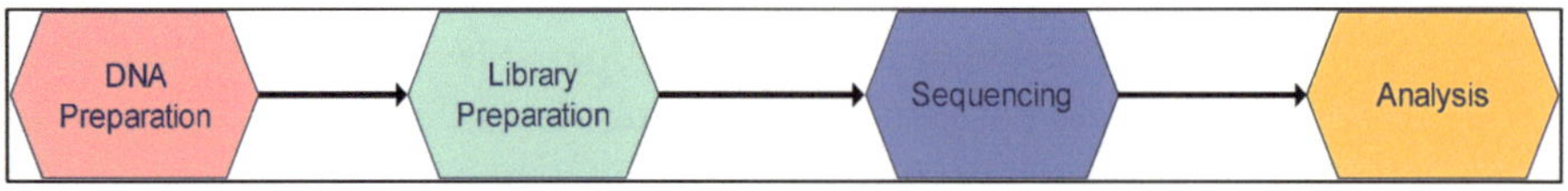

Figure 5.
Overview of DNA sequencing. DNA sequencing involves preparation of target DNA (sample collection and nucleic acid extraction); library preparation (adaptor ligation, size selection, and amplification); sequencing and data analysis (base calling, alignment, and annotation).

Tafenoquine is a single-dose (300 mg) drug approved only for use in combination with chloroquine (CQ) for adult patients who are nonpregnant and G-6-PD-normal. Before administering TQ, make sure the patient has normal G-6-PD activity (>70% [7, 61]. In pregnant or breastfeeding women, consider weekly chemoprophylaxis with CQ until delivery and breastfeeding is completed. Then, based on their G-6-PD status, treat with PQ to avoid future relapse [61].

4. Epidemiology of malaria recurrence

4.1 Prevalence of malaria recurrence

4.1.1 World

Malaria recurrence is a daunting public health problem worldwide. It increases the incidence and prevalence of malaria [9, 26, 60]. In many regions, a large portion of *P. vivax* prevalence is attributed to relapse [9, 16, 62]. A long-term study conducted on Thai-Myanmar border revealed a higher rate of *P. vivax* than *P. falciparum* recurrence, with a cumulative proportion of 31.5% (95% CI: 30.1–33.0%) and 21.5% (95% CI: 20.3–22.8%) recurrence by day 63, respectively [63].

In the recent meta-analysis by Hossain *et al.*, recurrent parasitemia of *Plasmodium* species between day 7 and 42 was documented among 13.2% of patients worldwide, mainly of *P. vivax* recurrence. In the same report, the cumulative risks of recurrent parasitemia of any *Plasmodium* species by day 28, 42, and 63 were 8.1% (95% CI: 7.7–8.6), 16.8% (95% CI: 16.2–17.5), and 30.5% (95% CI: 29.4–31.6), respectively [12]. Additionally, a comprehensive review involving many studies across Asia, the Americas, and Africa showed a recurrence of *P. vivax* in 30% of people within 2 months after ACT [64]. In India, a country with a high burden of *P. vivax* region, 17.1% average relapse rates of *P. vivax* with quickly recurring type have been recorded from 2001 to 2003 [65]. Likewise, in Brazil, 23% of reported cases of *P. vivax* malaria relapse [66].

Relapse persisted as the contributor to the overall prevalence of recurrent malaria worldwide. A genotyping and whole-genome sequencing conducted in Cambodia for assessing the efficacy of CQ against *P. vivax* indicated that two-thirds of the recurrent *P. vivax* parasites resulted from heterologous relapses [67]. The incidence density of *P. vivax* recurrence was 45.1/100 patient-years, mostly occurring between the 4th and 13th week after initiating treatment [66]. The cumulative incidence of the first recurrence of *P. vivax* infection among patients receiving CQ and PQ in Turbo Municipality, Colombia, was 24.1% (95% CI: 14.6–33.7%). The majority (65.5%) of these recurrences were classified as relapse and occurred within 51 to 110 days of follow-up. High genetic diversity (12.5%) of *P. vivax* strains was recorded in the area. In general, relapse from *P. vivax* infection is responsible for the majority of recurrent malaria [68].

Recrudescence, with its potential to reveal treatment failure, carries an essential implication for the effectiveness of malaria treatment [5]. Recrudescence of *P. falciparum* 13 years after exposure was reported from Liberia. This woman is 49 years old with no history of traveling outside Canada, and never received a blood transfusion [69]. Recrudescence of *P. falciparum* after 4 years in a Ghanian pregnant woman living in Italy raised a speculation on the role of pregnancy triggering too late recrudescence by impairing preexisting immunity. Additionally, after relocating from a malaria-endemic area to a nonendemic area, patients may lose their immunity and develop recrudescence of the chronic *P. falciparum* infection [70].

4.1.2 Sub-Saharan Africa

Given the quality of interventions, co-endemicity of parasites, and climatic conditions, recurrence remains a formidable problem in sub-Saharan Africa [71]. Recrudescence of *P. falciparum* 13 years after exposure of a woman was reported in Liberia. This woman was 49 years old with no history of traveling outside Canada and never received a blood transfusion [69]. In Malawi, nearly 30% of children treated for malaria are reinfected within 42 days of treatment [72]. Greater immunity to *P. vivax* was conferred by reinfection with homologous parasite strain than with heterologous parasite strain. This was indicated by a reduction in the geometric mean of parasite count and in fever episodes from primary infection to reinfection [73]. These findings reflect the remaining problem in sub-Saharan Africa despite progress in the twenty-first century [74].

4.1.3 Ethiopia

Ethiopia as a sub-Saharan African country with a 75% malarious landmass, where *P. falciparum* and *P. vivax* are co-endemic, suffers from multidimensional burden of malaria and its recurrence. The risk of malaria recurrence in Ethiopia by day 28 and day 42 was 2.8% (95% CI: 0.9–8.4%) and 6.7% (95% CI: 3.2–13.5%), respectively [75]. The risk of *P. vivax* infection following treatment with rapidly eliminated treatments needs attention. After radical cure of primary *P. vivax* infection with PQ and CQ, 0.4 *P. vivax* infections/person/year was reported from Ethiopia by Abreha *et al.* [76]. Assuming these all as reinfections and the potential of slowly eliminated ACTs, the expected risk of *P. vivax* recurrence by day 63, 3.8% incidence is estimated in Ethiopia [12].

Malaria recurrence is among important public health problems in Ethiopia. An open-label trial aimed to assess the effectiveness of artemether lumefantrine (AL) in Jimma Zone by Eshetu *et al.,* detected a 3.8% and 5.1% reinfection and recrudescence of *P. falciparum* by day 42, respectively. The same study identified a higher (9.4%) rate of *P. falciparum* recrudescence among children aged below 6 years in the Jimma zone. The lower capacity of children to sufficiently metabolize the drug has been suggested for the therapeutic yield [77]. Similarly, recurrent parasitemia rates of 19% and 7.5% after 28 days following treatment with AL and CQ, respectively, were observed in Ethiopia. This was considered as the incidence rate of treatment failure using *in vivo* parameters [78]. Furthermore, Teklehaimanot and his colleagues reported recurrent episodes of vivax malaria despite the use of an optimum dose of PQ and relocation of patients to a non-malarious area, from Gambella to Addis Ababa. This report alarms failure of PQ to prevent relapse in Ethiopia, where *P. vivax* is responsible for 40% of malaria prevalence (**Figure 6**) [79].

4.2 Factors affecting malaria recurrence

The recurrence of malaria depends upon various factors. These factors can be associated with the human host (gender, gene, and others), the *Plasmodium* parasite (specie, mono or mixed infection, and density), and intervention deployed (type of antimalarial drug) [12, 17, 80–82].

DOI: http://dx.doi.org/10.5772/intechopen.108888

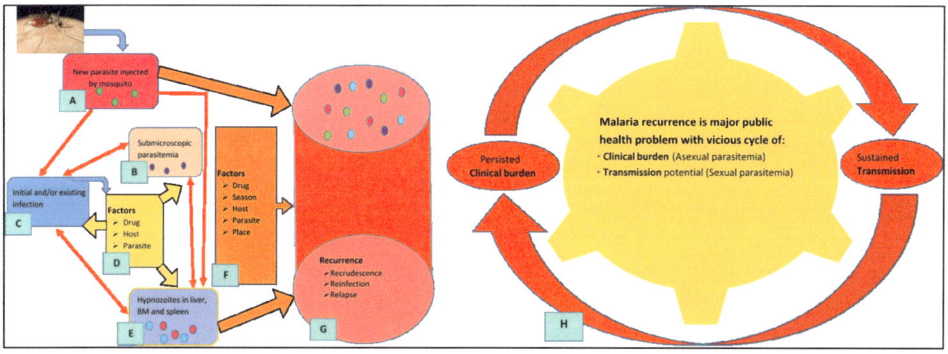

Figure 6.
Overview of malaria recurrence and its public health importance. Malaria recurrence can assume various forms depending upon the species of the plasmodium and other factors. (A) Primary infection due to inoculation of sporozoites by infected mosquito. (B) Sub-microscopic parasitemia is often missed by conventional diagnostic tools. (C) Infection with malaria parasites can be primary or recurrence. (D) Factors arising from the human host, the parasite, or intervention can determine the type of malaria recurrence. (E) Hypnozoites from the liver can give rise to recurrence or vice versa. (F) the prevalence of malaria recurrence depends on places, human hosts, type of drugs used, and season. (G) Recurrence is characterized by renewed parasitemia in peripheral circulation due to relapse, reinfection, or recrudescence. (H) Public health implication of malaria recurrence. Colored small circles: Green = new parasite injected as sporozoite, pale blue = hypnozoites from newly injected parasites, purple = existing parasites as sub-microscopic in the circulation, and red = long existing hypnozoite.

4.2.1 Human host factors

4.2.1.1 Genetic factors

The pattern of malaria recurrence, especially relapse, depends on host factors; including the cytochrome enzyme responsible for metabolizing anti-relapse drug. The prominent anti-relapse drug, PQ, is converted into its active metabolites in the liver by monoamine oxide and CYP2D6 (isotype of cytochrome P450 [CYP450]) enzymes [81]. CYP2D6 is naturally polymorphic, and its variant is widespread; up to 25% of the world's population. This variant is associated with a substantial decline in efficacy of PQ putting people with this variant gene at higher risk of relapse [82, 83]. The host immune efficiency to clear parasitemia during the initial infection is important for the possibility of future recurrence [17]. The risk of *P. vivax* recurrence among patients who failed to clear their initial parasitemia within 2 days (AHR = 1.8 95% CI: 1.4–2.3; $P < 0.001$) [12]. People with a deficiency of the G-6-PD enzyme, owing to their ineligibility to PQ and TQ, carry a higher risk of vivax malaria recurrence [9, 61]. Pregnant and those breastfeeding children below 6 months, G-6-PD-deficient individuals, and children below 6 months do not receive PQ, and hence are at risk of recurrence [84, 85]. Also, according to a mathematical modeling study in Brazil, once infected with *P. vivax*, 23% of pregnant women are at risk of one or more episodes of vivax recurrence within 3 months [86]. Another modeling result shows the rise in *P. vivax* recurrence with an increase in the proportion of people with G-6-PD deficiency in the population [26].

4.2.1.2 Age

Being at a younger age raised the risk of *P. vivax* infection recurrence in the Thai-Myanmar border ($P = 0.001$) [63]. Patients with younger age (AHR = 3.04 95% CI: 2.39–3.87, $P < 0.001$) carry a greater risk of developing recurrent *P. vivax* parasitemia than adults [12]. Likewise, Antonio *et al*. 2021, recently reported a higher frequency of malaria recurrences among children under 4 years [87]. Slow clearance of parasites due to dose variation by age and weight; and subtherapeutic dose due to manipulation to overcome the bitter taste of drugs, particularly CQ, are some of the factors that are suggested to escalate the frequency of recurrence among children [87–89].

4.2.1.3 Gender

Male gender increased the risk of recurrence during the year in Brazil and Thailand [62, 63, 66]. Male patients (AHR = 1.26 95% CI: 1.08–1.46; P = 0.003) carry a greater risk of developing recurrent *P. vivax* [12]. This might be due to the behavior of the male that exposes him to a new infection with *P. falciparum*, which in turn triggers relapse. Additionally, more proportion of males is not eligible for PQ than females, which might raise the risk [12, 80, 90].

4.2.2 Parasite factor

Parasite-related factors, such as species, strain, density, and stage, play a fundamental role in the pattern of malaria recurrence [9].

4.2.2.1 Species

Species of the offending parasite are the leading factors driving malaria recurrence. *P. vivax* is responsible for the majority of recurrent malaria [9, 87]. A long-term study conducted on Thai-Myanmar border, revealed a higher frequency of *P. vivax* than *P. falciparum* recurrence, with a cumulative proportion of 31.5% (95% CI: 30.1–33.0%) and 21.5% (95% CI: 20.3–22.8%) recurrence by day 63, respectively [63]. Similarly, other supportive findings show the contribution of *P. vivax* for at least 70% of malaria recurrences [12, 62].

4.2.2.2 Density

The density of parasites, mainly the load of asexual parasites in the peripheral circulation enhances recurrence, particularly recrudescence, by giving resilience to the dose of treatment. Higher parasitemia and a shorter time since the onset of symptoms in the initial infection increased the risk of relapse during the year in Brazil and the Thai-Myanmar border [63, 66]. A similar effect of hyperparasitemia on severe recrudescence was observed in France, where a polyclonal infection and high load of parasites increased the risk in a participant, who returned from Chad [91]. On the other hand, patients with high parasite count (AHR = 1.59 95% CI: 1.22–2.08; P = 0.001), carry a greater risk of developing recurrent *P. vivax* [12]. Furthermore, according to a modeling study, individuals with more hypnozoites are predicted to experience more relapses [60].

4.2.2.3 Mixed-infection

In areas, where *P. falciparum* and *P. vivax* malaria are co-endemic, patients treated for *P. falciparum* infection have a high risk of subsequent *P. vivax* malaria. According to Commons *et al.*, the risk of *P. vivax* parasitemia after *P. falciparum* at day 63 was 24% [12]. A series of RCTs in Thai-Myanmar revealed that a mixed infection and

P. falciparum gametocytemia at enrollment raised the risk of *P. vivax* recurrence (P = 0.001) [63]. Similar other studies indicated the increased risk of relapse of *P. vivax* after infection with *P. falciparum* [80]. This suggests the potential role of *P. falciparum* infection to trigger the dormant *P. vivax* [12, 80]. Due to the suppression by *P. falciparum*, *P. vivax* disappears from the blood without reaching a density that can elicit a host immune response. Taking this defeat as a chance or tactic, *P. vivax* reemerges after weeks or months by generating transmissible densities of gametocytes. Besides, in low transmission settings, when immunity to *P. falciparum* is weak, falciparum malaria in adults may trigger dormant hypnozoites of *P. vivax* due to its capacity to trigger fever [20].

The growing pieces of evidence from all over the world about the correlation between the risks of *P. vivax* after *P. falciparum* treatment raise curiosity that the immune response of the host to acute malaria might trigger the revival of *P. vivax* hypnozoites. Besides, although the exact mechanism remains unclear, fever and hemolysis in *P. falciparum* infection are the suggested triggers for relapse [12, 80]. According to the report of the study in Thailand by Douglas *et al.*, 51% of patients diagnosed with acute infection of *P. falciparum* and treated with a rapidly eliminated drug suffered a relapse of *P. vivax* after just 2 months [63]. Furthermore, a meta-analysis of clinical trials on *P. falciparum* by Commons *et al.* demonstrated that within 63 days, 24% of *P. falciparum* patients suffered from a *P. vivax* recurrence. This review reported that nearly 70% of malaria recurrences are due to *P. vivax* [12]. Taken together, these shreds of evidence not only show the sizeable input of relapse to the general epidemiology of malaria but also demonstrate how relapse wisely uses the inoculated sporozoites to optimize the survival of these species [11, 20].

4.2.3 Intervention-related and other factors

4.2.3.1 Drug

Drugs are profound determinants of malaria recurrence [63]. According to a series of clinical trials conducted for nearly 15 years on the Thai-Myanmar border, recurrence of *P. vivax* infection after 63 days was higher by 3.6 to 4.2-fold among participants treated with artemether-lumefantrine and artesunate-atovaquone-proguanil combinations compared to those treated with artemisinin-based combinations involving mefloquine or piperaquine [63].

ACTs containing mefloquine or piperaquine are better than ACTs containing AL at delaying the risk of recurrence. However, time-dependent efficacy decline has been revealed by a systematic review that reported a 15% prevalence of *P. vivax* recurrence among ACT recipients after day 63. The risk of *P. vivax* recurrence raises with the number of days after any antimalarial treatment given for *P. falciparum* infection [12]. Also, artesunate monotherapy may lead to recrudescence of parasitemia in 40–50% of cases within 28 days owing to drug-induced dormancy [92]. A comparable result has been observed in France, on a patient who returned from Chad [91].

Slowly eliminated antimalarials reduce the likelihood of early recurrence. Douglas *et al.* reported that the cumulative risk of *P. vivax* recurrence secondary to *P. falciparum* mono-infection was 51.1% after treatment with rapidly eliminated drugs (t1/2 < 1 day), 35.3% after treatment with intermediate half-life drugs (t1/2 1–7 days), and 19.6% after treatment with slowly eliminated drugs (t1/2 > 7 days) (P < 0.001) by day 63 [63]. Consistently, the risk of recurrence was higher for AL than for DHA-PPQ therapy. The proposed reason is the shorter dormancy of parasitemia for rapidly eliminated drugs, such as lumefantrine, in AL [12, 93].

Incorporating PQ, hypnozoiticidal drug, in standard malaria drugs reduces the risk of recurrence, particularly relapse. Primaquine, when combined with ACT and PQ, can reduce the risk of recurrence in *P. vivax* and *P. falciparum* co-endemic settings [12]. Consistent with this, PQ combined with either CQ or AL has reduced the recurrence of *P. vivax* infection among G-6-PD wild patients by 5-fold for 1 year in Ethiopia [76]. Considering a one-year-long RCT in Thailand, a high dose of PQ (7 mg/kg) over 7 or 14 days is efficacious in preventing *P. vivax* relapse. Similarly, at least one episode of *P. vivax* recurrence has occurred among 70% of subjects in non-PQ arms compared to 18% of subjects in the PQ arm [15].

According to a systematic review by Commons *et al.*, the risk of *P. vivax* recurrence with a lower dose of CQ was 32.4% (95% CI: 29.8–35.1) by day 42. However, raising the dose substantially reduced the risk. Furthermore, including PQ in the treatment significantly reduced the risk of recurrence by day 42 from (AHR = 0.82 95% CI: 0.69–0.97; P = 0.021) with CQ alone to (AHR = 0.10, 0.05–0.17; P < 0.0001) with CQ and PQ. This strengthens the concept of the role of PQ as a radical cure in effectively preventing the early recurrence of *P. vivax* [89]. Nevertheless, despite the renowned efficacy of PQ, few pieces of evidence are emerging on malaria recurrence after radical therapy. Considering the tests, they used microscopy and the unknown status of CYP2D6, these pieces of evidence reflect treatment failure, but do not confirm drug resistance [79]. After its introduction, ACT rendered the rate of recrudescence to be below 10% in Jimma zone, southwest Ethiopia [77]. It is strongly considered that the probability of artemisinin resistance with a standard dose, a 3 day ACT, is rare if the proportion of day 3 positive smears is below 3% [94].

4.2.3.2 Place

In co-endemic locations, patients presenting with *P. falciparum* are highly likely to carry *P. vivax* hypnozoites that give rise to recurrence [12, 80]. Patients in regions of short relapse periodicity had a greater rate of *P. vivax* parasitemia than those in regions of long periodicity (HR = 8.61 95% CI: 2.34–31.65; P = 0.001) [12]. Also, the risk of *P. vivax* parasitemia was 6.5% (95% CI: 4.6–8.6) in regions of short periodicity compared with 1.9% (95% CI: 0.4–4.0) in areas of long periodicity [12, 17]. Therefore, geographical variation determines the frequency of malaria recurrence.

4.2.3.3 Season

A dormant hypnozoite of *P. vivax* awaits the right time for activation to take evolutionary advantage, thereby ensuring maximum likelihood of transmission and immune evasion. To ensure optimum transmission, hypnozoites synchronize their wake-up time to a season with an abundant mosquito population [20]. Thus, the incidence of symptomatic malaria was higher in September (OR = 2.81 95% CI: 2.1–3.7) and October (OR = 2.4 95% CI: 1.8–3.2) than in November [95].

5. Recurrence and malaria transmission

Malaria recurrence, in addition to rising clinical episodes, increases the probability of malaria transmission. In fact, all types of malaria recurrence increase transmission in multidimensional ways, including by raising longevity of infectiousness and transmission potential [6, 11, 20]. A systematic review and meta-analysis result revealed that recrudescent (AOR = 9.05 95% CI: 3.74–21.9) and reinfection (AOR = 3.03 95% CI: 1.66–5.54) with *P. falciparum* were strongly associated with gametocytemia after day 7 [29]. Hence, recurrent infections with *Plasmodium* species maintain the potential for malaria transmission [6, 9, 16].

Recurring malaria leads to erythrocytic schizogony that renews or escalates peripheral parasitemia. Such parasitemia entails gametocytogenesis that maintains the transmission of malaria, thereby complicating elimination and eradication efforts [6, 16, 96, 97]. Moreover, activation of hypnozoites from different earlier inoculations can produce at least two genotypes simultaneously growing inside the patient's blood. This produces genetically distinct gametocytes that, if taken by a mosquito, have a high probability to undergo meiotic recombination resulting in genetic variation. This phenomenon is considered as a major factor for high degree

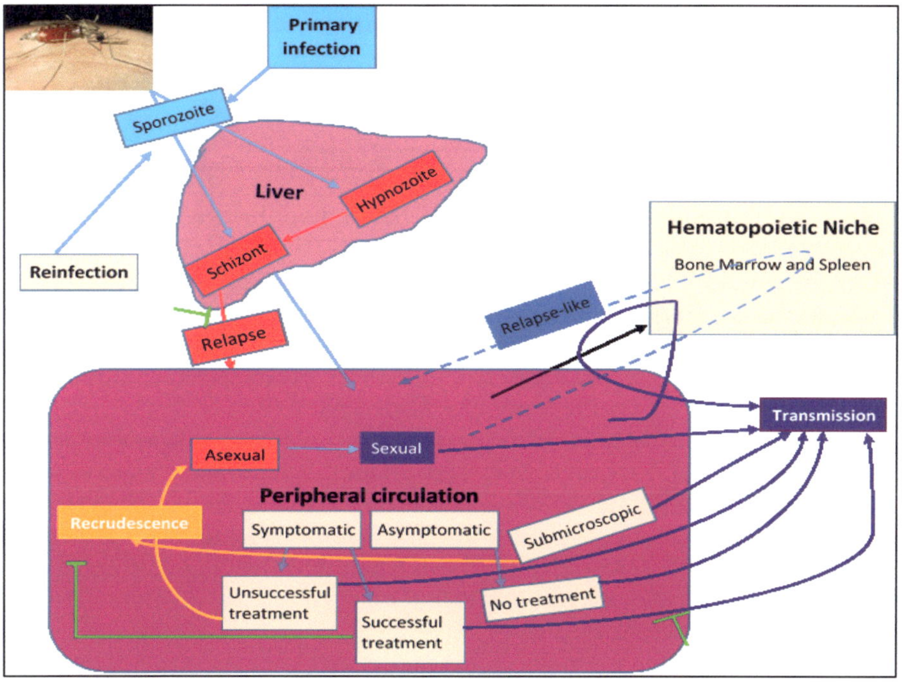

Figure 7.
Pattern of malaria recurrence, spots to intervene, and its prevention strategies. Parasitemia in peripheral circulation can be due to symptomatic, asymptomatic, or sub-microscopic plasmodium infection. This peripheral parasitemia can also arise from any type of malaria recurrence. (red boxes): After arriving in the liver, the inoculated sporozoites either transform into schizonts or directly become hypnozoites that later can become schizonts. Schizonts arising from latent hypnozoites or the inoculated sporozoites release merozoites that join the blood circulation to eventually produce asexual parasites. (purple boxes and lines): Young gametocytes localize into the hematopoietic niche and rejoin the circulation when reach stage five gametocyte. Gametocytes can result from unsuccessful treatment, after successful treatment with non-gametocidal drugs, and any untreated infection. These gametocytes mediate the transmission of malaria. (broken blue lines): Asexual parasites that periodically sequester in the hematopoietic niche and return into circulation resulting in relapse-like parasitemia. (blue solid lines): Flow of malaria pathogenesis from primary and reinfection subsequent to inoculation of sporozoites. (black line): Parasites sequestering in the hematopoietic niche. (greenish-yellow box and lines): Unsuccessful treatment and sub-microscopic infections give rise to recrudescence and/or possible transmission. (Green lines): Possible weak points for intervention (such as prompt diagnosis and effective treatment with efficacious radical cure, and transmission-blocker) to tackle recurrence and/or transmission.

of genetic diversity seen in *P. vivax* over settings with very low seasonal transmission [17]. Hence, recurrence confers *P. vivax* with maximum opportunity for transmission and immune evasion [20].

Recurrence of *P. vivax* worsens transmission of malaria with its potential to promptly produce gametocytes and transmit before treatment initiation. In addition, due to the continued reactivation of hypnozoite, the patient remains a potential reservoir of infection for a long time from just a single inoculum [9, 97]. The probability of relapse and subsequent transmission raises with a load of hypnozoite in the liver [6, 60]. Furthermore, if the recurrence involves a heterologous genotype, it paves the ways for the development of drug resistance, thereby transmission of variant species. The variant species together with other factors cause recrudescence, which expands the pool of recurrence, and the subsequent transmission [20]. Besides, reinfection further exacerbates transmission dynamics with its potential to activate hypnozoite; introduce a new strain unresponsive to therapy and provides an opportunity for immune evasion [11].

Generally, malaria recurrence sustains and/or intensifies transmission. It raises efficiency, chance, and longevity of transmission, thus threatening the success of interventions [11]. Thus, it is wise to consider fighting recurrence to break transmission and eliminate malaria (**Figure** 7) [60, 96–98].

6. Recurrence and malaria elimination strategies

The axiom "prevention is better than cure" better describes the impact of recurrence on the efforts to eliminate malaria [9, 85]. The difficulty to diagnose and treat malaria substantially increases morbidity and mortality among patients. Relapse due to vivax malaria is refractory to the majority of the current treatments since the sole hypnozoiticidal-drug, PQ, is challenged by many factors [9, 20]. The use of ACT will more noticeably reduce the prevalence of *P. falciparum* prevalence than *P. vivax* due to its inability to kill the hypnozoite forms of *P. vivax* [19].

A relapse followed by asymptomatic parasitemia could be the major approach to *P. vivax* transmission [20]. Particularly recurrence from asymptomatic infections is the major challenge to the elimination of malaria as they arrive at the gametocyte stage at the level below the sensitivity of the current gold standard tool for malaria diagnosis: light microscopy [9, 17]. Asymptomatic *P. vivax* infections are common in malaria-endemic locations [36]. However, the contribution of relapse for asymptomatic malaria is not well known [9, 16, 19].

Vivax malaria remained the major global challenge despite a spectacular achievement against *P. falciparum* [74]. The complex nature of *P. vivax*, mainly due to relapse, extensively wrinkled the effectiveness of the radical cure with PQ. A considerable portion of the global population has difficulty converting PQ into its active form, hence the increased risk of recurrence [9]. Pregnant women and children below 6 months old owing to their ineligibility to PQ are at risk of vivax malaria and its recurrence. They can also serve as potential human reservoirs of infection [9, 85]. Hence, it is prevention that helps to keep this ever-complicating parasite at its bay [9, 16, 17, 99].

The possibility of relapse secondary to treatment and/or immunologic response to *P. falciparum* infection perpetuates the transmission in co-endemic settings. The growing phenomena of resistance to antimalarials, such as CQ and ACT, is another fuel to recurrence. The ineligibility of the vast majority of population to PQ given their physiological and genetic condition places a hurdle on the stride toward preventing recurrence [9].

The frequent possibility of mutation in *P. vivax* owing to cross-reactivity between strain arising from hypnozoite and strain from mosquito in an environment challenges the efficacy of therapies [14, 17]. Different intervals of recurrence resulting from the variation of *P. vivax* population in tropics (frequent relapse) and temperate (long latency) regions is another nightmare. Moreover, the capacity to remain sub-clinical and submicroscopic with huge potential to quickly produce gametocytes offers the cutting-edge to this parasite triumph [11, 17, 20, 100].

In general, the recurrence of *Plasmodium* infection, especially the *P. vivax* relapse, is the major setback to malaria elimination strategies of the time. Consequently, there is a renewed focus on *P. vivax* due to the mounting accumulation of evidence on the maliciousness of vivax malaria [9]. To achieve malaria eradication goal, we must consider all species of *Plasmodium*; while improving the transmission-reducing potential of interventions [6, 14, 19]. It is key to underpin prevention mainly for infants and pregnant women, while keeping the search for targets of intervention to stay in the game [9].

7. Conclusion and future remarks

Malaria recurrence plays a considerable part in sustaining malaria epidemiology. Understanding the biology and epidemiology of malaria recurrence is crucial to overcome current challenges to efforts in malaria elimination. Malaria recurrence is not adequately studied partly due to the complex nature of the disease and logistic constraints for diagnosis. Regardless of its role in complicating clinical and public health impact of malaria, a basic understanding of malaria recurrence is limited. In this review, we have discussed the biology and epidemiology of malaria recurrence along with its implication on malaria mitigation.

Recurring malaria leads to increased morbidity and mortality due to malaria. By creating opportunities for gametocytogenesis, it sustains malaria transmission. Without identifying the specific *Plasmodium* species responsible for recurrence in specific areas limits the effectiveness of interventions. Lack of clear idea about the specific type of recurrence raises misconception on drug efficacy that eventually leads to hasty prohibition of antimalarials without robust replacement. Without effective intervention based on a clear understanding of recurrent malaria, morbidity and mortality continue to escalate due to recurrence. Unmanaged recurrent malaria maintains transmission of malaria. Hence, failure to promptly deal with recurrent malaria in a certain area has a huge impact on the health of individuals and the community at large.

Due to its widespread prevalence, relapse propensity, complex process of diagnosis and treatment, as well as other aspects, *P. vivax* demands continued multidimensional research. Studies should focus on the biology of malaria recurrence to improve the yield of control interventions. Optimizing disease-control interventions prevent a recurrence and breaks transmission to eliminate malaria.

8. Outstanding questions

1. How to detect and quantify *P. vivax* hypnozoite?

2. How much is the contribution of relapse for asymptomatic malaria?

3. How to detect and identify markers to characterize three types of recurrence in vivax malaria?

4. How to differentiate non-hypnozoite-driven and non-bloodstream-originating relapse?

5. How can we measure the contribution of the hematopoietic niche to malaria recurrence?

6. What is the frequency of malaria recurrence among the "PQ-hard-to-reach population," particularly in settings where *P. falciparum* and *P. vivax* are co-endemic?

7. How can we measure/model the contribution of the "PQ-hard-to-reach populations" to the overall transmission potential?

8. How can we improve the prevention and control of malaria among the most vulnerable, but "PQ-hard-to-reach population?"

9. After how many recurrences will a new drug-resistant strain/species develop? and does it depend on species?

10. How much of reinfection with *P. vivax* will remain asymptomatic in mixed infection (*P. falciparum* + *P. vivax*)?

11. What is the pattern of recurrence by mono-infection and mixed-infection?

12. What proportion of mixed infection (*P. falciparum* + *P. vivax*) is properly treated and/or miss-treated as *P. falciparum* single infection?

13. How can we differentiate non-hypnozoite-originating relapse from true relapse?

9. Search strategy and selection criteria

We searched PubMed, the Cochrane Library, Science Direct, and Google Scholar for articles published in English between January 01, 2000, and December 31, 2021, with the terms "malaria recurrence," "malaria relapse," "malaria reinfection," "*Plasmodium* vivax," "recurrent parasitemia," "malaria recrudescence" and combined with the terms "glucose-six-phosphate dehydrogenase, "primaquine." We also included review studies (published between January 01, 2000, and December 31, 2021) cited by articles identified by this search strategy and selected those we identified as relevant. Selected review articles are cited to provide readers with more details and references than this review can accommodate.

Acknowledgements

The author is grateful to Mr. Wasihun Admassu for his important comments on the first draft of this paper. The author also thanks Mr. Ahmed Kamil for his help in the drawing process of diagrams.

Author's contributions

AA has conceived and designed this review. AA has participated in the acquisition of data and preparation of the draft manuscript. AA is involved in drafting, critically reviewing, and final approval of this manuscript.

Abbreviations

ACT	artemisinin combination therapy
AHR	adjusted hazard ratio
AL	artemether lumefantrine
CI	confidence interval
CQ	chloroquine
CYP450	cytochrome P450
DNA	de-oxy ribonucleic acid
DHA-PPQ	dihydro-artimesinine piperaquine
GLURP	glutamate rich protein
G-6-PD	glucose six phosphate dehydrogenase
MSP	merozoite surface protein
nPCR	nested polymerase chain reaction
OR	odds ratio
PCR	polymerase chain reaction
PQ	premaquine
qPCR	quantitative polymerase chain reaction
rRNA	ribosomal ribonucleic acid
TQ	tafenoquine

Author details

Aklilu Alemayehu[1,2]

1 School of Medical Laboratory Sciences, Institute of Health, Jimma University, Jimma, Ethiopia

2 Department of Medical Laboratory Sciences, College of Medicine and Health Sciences, Arba Minch University, Arba Minch, Ethiopia

*Address all correspondence to: aaakealex59@gmail.com

References

[1] World Health Organization. Global Malaria Programme. WHO Malaria Terminology. Geneva: WHO; 2019

[2] Encyclopedia of Malaria. New York: Springer Science+Business Media; 2013

[3] Marcus MB. The hypnozoite concept, with particular reference to malaria. Parasitology Research. 2011;**108**:247-252

[4] *P. vivax* Information Hub. Knowledge sharing for Relapsing Malaria. Focus on: Relapse, Reinfection or Recrudescence. 2021. Available from: www.vivaxmalaria.org

[5] World Health Organization. Medicines for Malaria Venture. Methods and techniques for clinical trials on antimalarial drug efficacy: Genotyping to identify parasite populations. In: Informal Consultation Organized by the Medicines for Malaria Venture and Cosponsored by the World Health Organization. Amesterdam: WHO; 2008

[6] Markus MB. Biological concepts in recurrent *P. vivax* malaria. Parasitology. 2018;**143**(13):1-7

[7] World Health Organization Global Malaria Programme. Report on Antimalarial Drug Efficacy, Resistance and Response: 10 Years of Surveillance (2010-2019). Geneva: WHO; 2020

[8] World Health Organization. WHO Guidelines for Malaria. Geneva: WHO; 2021

[9] Baird JK. Malaria caused by *P. vivax*: Recurrent, difficult to treat, disabling, and threatening to life- averting the infectious bite preempts these hazards. Pathogens and Global Health. 2013;**107**(8):475-479

[10] Lau YL, Tan LH, Chin LC, Fong MY, Noraishah MA, Rohela M. *P. knowlesi* reinfection in human. Emerging Infectious Diseases. 2011;**17**(7):1314

[11] Águas R, Ferreira MU, Gomes MGM. Modeling the effects of relapse in the transmission dynamics of malaria parasites. Journal of Parasitology Research. 2012;**2012**:1-15

[12] Commons RJ, Ja S, Thriemer K, Hossain MS, Douglas NM, Humphreys GS, et al. Risk of *P. vivax* parasitemia after *P. falciparum* infection: A systematic review and meta-analysis. The Lancet Infectious Diseases. 2019;**19**(1):91-101

[13] White NJ. How antimalarial drug resistance affects post-treatment prophylaxis. Malaria Journal. 2008;**7**(9):1-7

[14] McCann RS, Cohee LM, Goupeyou-Youmsi J, Laufer MK. Maximizing impact: Can interventions to prevent clinical malaria reduce parasite transmission? Trends in Parasitology. 2020;**36**(11):906-913

[15] Chu C. Management of relapsing *P. vivax* malaria. International Journal of Infectious Diseases. 2016;**45**:16

[16] Markus MB. Malaria eradication and the hidden parasite reservoir. Trends in Parasitology. 2017;**33**(7):492-495

[17] White NJ. Determinants of relapse periodicity in *P. vivax* malaria. Malaria Journal. 2011;**10**(297):1-36

[18] Brasil P, Costa ADP, Pedro RS, Bressan CS, Silva S, Tauil PL, et al. Unexpectedly long incubation period of *P. vivax* malaria, in the absence of chemoprophylaxis, in patients diagnosed

outside the transmission area in Brazil. Malaria Journal. 2011;**10**(122):1-5

[19] World Health Organization. Confronting *P. vivax* Malaria. Geneva: WHO; 2015

[20] White NJ. Why do some primate malarias relapse? Trends in Parasitology. 2016;**32**(12):918-920

[21] Obaldia N III, Meibalan E, Sa JM, Ma S, Clark MA, Mejia P, et al. Bone marrow is a major parasite reservoir in *P. vivax* infection. MBio. 2018;**9**(3):e00625-e00618

[22] Markus MB. New evidence for Hypnozoite-Independent *P. vivax* malarial recurrences. Trends in Parasitology. 2018;**34**(12):1015-1016

[23] Silva-Filho JL, Lacerda MVG, Recker M, Wassmer SC, Marti M, Costa FTM. *P. vivax* in hematopoietic niches: Hidden and dangerous. Trends in Parasitology. 2020;**36**(5):447-458

[24] Bright AT, Tewhey R, Arango EM, Wang T, Schork NJ, et al. A high-resolution case study of a patient with recurrent *P. vivax* infections shows that relapses were caused by meiotic siblings. PLOS Neglected Tropical Disease. 2014;**8**(6):e2882

[25] Battle KEKM, Bhatt S, Gething PW, Howes RE, Golding N, et al. Geographical variation in *P. vivax* relapse. Malaria Journal. 2014;**13**(144):1-16

[26] Chamchod F, Beier JC. Modeling *P. vivax*: Relapses, treatment, seasonality, and G6PD deficiency. Journal of Theoretical Biology. 2013;**316**:25-34

[27] Mueller I, Galinski MR, P JKB, Carlton JM, Kochar DK, Alonso PL, et al. Key gaps in knowledge of *P. vivax*, a neglected human malaria parasite. The Lancet Infectious Diseases. 2009;**9**(9):555-566

[28] Witkowski B, Khim N, Chim P, Kim S, Ke S, Kloeung N, et al. Reduced artemisinin susceptibility of *P. falciparum* ring stages in western Cambodia. Antimicrobial Agents and Chemotherapy. 2013;**57**:914-923

[29] Abdulla S, Achan J, Adam I, Alemayehu BH, Allan R, Allen EN, et al. Gametocyte carriage in uncomplicated *P. falciparum* malaria following treatment with artemisinin combination therapy: A systematic review and meta-analysis of individual patient data. BMC Medicine. 2016;**14**(1):1-18

[30] Cheng Z. Advances in molecular diagnosis of malaria. In: Makowski G, editor. Adv Clin Chem. 80: Academic Press; 2017

[31] World Health Organization. Global Technical Strategy for Malaria 2016-2030. Geneva: WHO; 2015

[32] Tedla M. A focus on improving molecular diagnostic approaches to malaria control and elimination in low transmission settings: Review. Parasite Epidemiology and Control. 2019;**6**:e00107

[33] Snounou G, Singh B. Nested PCR analysis of *plasmodium* parasites. In: Doolan DL, Editor. Methods Mol Med. 72. Totowa: Humana Press; 2002

[34] Hemingway J, Shretta R, Wells TNC, Bell D, Djimdé A, Achee N, et al. Tools and strategies for malaria control and elimination: What do we need to achieve a grand convergence in malaria? PLoS Biology. 2016;**14**(3):e1002380

[35] Green MR, Sambrook J. Nested Polymerase Chain Reaction (PCR). Huntington: Cold Spring Harbor Laboratory Press; 2019

[36] Assefa A, Ahmed AA, Deressa W, Wilson GG, Kebede A, Mohammed H, et al. Assessment of subpatent *plasmodium* infection in northwestern Ethiopia. Malaria Journal. 2020;**19**(108):1-10

[37] World Health Organization. Testing for G6PD Deficiency for Safe Use of Primaquine in Radical Cure of *P. Vivax* and *P. ovale* Malaria: Policy Brief. Geneva: WHO; 2016

[38] Canier L, Khim N, Kim S, Sluydts V, Heng S, Dourng D, et al. An innovative tool for moving malaria PCR detection of parasite reservoir into the field. Malaria Journal. 2013;**12**(405):1-12

[39] Perandin F. Development of a real-time PCR assay for detection of *P. falciparum, P. vivax, and P. ova*le for routine clinical diagnosis. Journal of Clinical Microbiology. 2004;**42**(3):1214-1219

[40] Rubio J, Benito A, Roche J, Berzosa P, Garcia M, Mico M, et al. Semi-nested, multiplex polymerase chain reaction for detection of human malaria parasites and evidence of *P. vivax* infection in Equatorial Guinea. American Journal of Tropical Medicine and Hygiene. 1999;**60**:183-187

[41] Thermo Fisher Scientific. Real-Time PCR Handbook 2021 [cited 2021 22/12/2021]. Available from: https://www.thermofisher.com/qpcr

[42] Kralik P, Ricchi M, Donu D. A basic guide to real time PCR in microbial diagnostics: Definitions, parameters, and everything. Frontiers in Microbiology. 2017;**8**(108):1-15

[43] Nsanzabana C, Djalle D, Guerin PJ, Menard D, Gonzalez IJ. Tools for surveillance of antimalarial-drug resistance: An assessment of current landascape. Malaria Journal. 2018;**17**(75):1-16

[44] Haanshuus CG, Mørch K, Blomberg B, Strøm GEA, Langeland N, Hanevik K, et al. Assessment of malaria real-time PCR methods and application with focus on lowlevel parasitaemia. PLoS One. 2019;**14**(7):1-15

[45] Leski TA, Taitt CR, Swaray AG, Bangura U, Reynolds ND, Holtz A, et al. Use of real-time multiplex PCR, malaria rapid diagnostic test and microscopy to investigate the prevalence of *plasmodium* species among febrile hospital patients in Sierra Leone. Malaria Journal. 2020;**19**(84):1-8

[46] Genomics F. What is Multiplex PCR? 2021. Available from: https://frontlinegenomics.com/what-is-multiplex-pcr/.

[47] Malaria Methods and Protocols. Doolan DL, editor. Totowa, New Jersey: Humana Press; 2017

[48] Gardner MJ, Hall N, Fung E, White O, Berriman M, Hyman RW, et al. Genome sequence of the human malaria parasite *plasmodium* falciparum. Nature Biotechnology. 2002;**419**:398-411

[49] Siegel SV, Rayner JC. Single cell sequencing shines a light on malaria parasite elatedness in complex infections. Trends in Parasitology. 2020;**36**(2):83-85

[50] Ford A, Kepple D, Abagero BR, Connors J, Pearson R, Auburn S, et al. Whole genome sequencing of *P. vivax* isolates reveals frequent sequence and structural polymorphisms in erythrocyte binding genes. PLoS Neglected Tropical Diseases. 2020;**14**(10):1-27

[51] Menard D, Chan ER, Benedet C, Ratsimbasoa A, Kim S, Chim P, et al. Whole genome sequencing of field isolates reveals a common duplication of the Duffy binding protein gene in

Malagasy *plasmodium* vivax strains. PLoS Neglected Tropical Diseases. 2013;7(11):1-15

[52] The malERA refresh consultative panel on Characterising the reservoir and measuring transmission malERA. An updated research agenda for characterising the reservoir and measuring transmission in malaria elimination and eradication. PLoS Medicine. 2017;**14**(11):e1002452

[53] Boussaroque A, Fall B, Madamet M, Camara C, Benoit N, Mansour FG, et al. Emergence of mutations in the K13 propeller gene of *P. falciparum* isolates from Dakar, Senegal, in 2013-2014. Antimicrobial Agents and Chemotherapy. 2016;**60**(1):624-627

[54] Heuchert A, Abduselam N, Zeynudin A, Eshetu T, Löscher T, Wieser A, et al. Molecular markers of anti-malarial drug resistance in Southwest Ethiopia over time: Regional surveillance from 2006 to 2013. Malaria Journal. 2015;**14**(1):1-7

[55] Tessema SK, Raman J, Duffy CW, Ishengoma DS, Amambua-Ngwa A, Greenhouse B. Applying next-generation sequencing to track falciparum malaria in sub-Saharan Africa. Malaria Journal. 2019;**18**(1):1-9

[56] Anjum MU, Naveed AK, Mahmood SN, Naveed OK. Single dose tafenoquine for preventing relapse in people with *P. vivax* malaria-an updated meta-analysis. Travel Medicine and Infectious Diseases. 2020;**36**(October 2019):101576

[57] Price RN, Commons RJ, Battle KE, Thriemer K, Mendis K. *P. Vivax* in the era of the shrinking *P. falciparum* map. Trends in Parasitology. 2020;**36**(6):560-570

[58] Robinson LJ, Wampfler R, Betuela I, Karl S, White MT, Suen CSLW. Strategies for understanding and reducing the *P. vivax* and *P. ovale* hypnozoite reservoir in Papua new Guinean children: A randomized placebo controlled trial and mathematical model. PLOS Medicine. 2015;**12**:e1001891

[59] Dini S, Douglas NM, Poespoprodjo JR, Kenangalem E, Sugiarto P, Plumb ID, et al. The risk of morbidity and mortality following recurrent malaria in Papua, Indonesia: A retrospective cohort study. BMC Medicine. 2020;**18**(28):1-12

[60] White MT, Karl S, Battle KE, Hay SI, Mueller I, Ghani AC. Modelling the contribution of the hypnozoite reservoir to *P. vivax* transmission. eLife. 2014;**3**:e04692

[61] World Health Organization. Control and Elimination of *P. Vivax* Malaria- a Technical Brief. Geneva: WHO; 2015

[62] Lawpoolsri S, Sattabongkot J, Sirichaisinthop J, Cui L, Kiattibutr K, Rachaphaew N, et al. Epidemiological profiles of recurrent malaria episodes in an endemic area along the Thailand-Myanmar border: A prospective cohort study. Malaria Journal. 2019;**18**(1):1-11

[63] Douglas NM, Nosten F, Ea A, Phaiphun L, Van Vugt M, Singhasivanon P, et al. *P. vivax* recurrence following falciparum and mixed species malaria: Risk factors and effect of antimalarial kinetics. Clinical Infectious Diseases. 2011;**52**(5):612-620

[64] Worldwide Antimalarial Resistance Network. A high risk of *P. vivax* after *P. falciparum* infection. 2019

[65] Ma S, Wajihullah SMI, Al-Khalifa MS. Malaria: Patterns of relapse and resistance. Journal of King Saud University- Science. 2010;**22**(1):31-36

[66] Simões LR, Alves ER, Ribatski-Silva D, Gomes LT, Nery AF, Fontes CJF. Factors associated with recurrent *P. vivax* malaria in Porto Velho, Rondônia state, Brazil, 2009. Cadernos de Saúde Pública. 2014;**30**(7):1403-1417

[67] Popovici J, Pierce-Friedrich L, Kim S, Bin S, Run V, Lek D, et al. Recrudescence, reinfection, or relapse? A more rigorous framework to assess chloroquine efficacy for *P. vivax* malaria. Journal of Infectious Diseases. 2019;**219**(2):315-322

[68] Zuluaga-Idárraga L, Blair S, Okoth SA, Udhayakumar V, Marcet PL, Aa E, et al. Prospective study of *P. vivax* malaria recurrence after radical treatment with a chloroquine-primaquine standard regimen in turbo, Colombia. Antimicrobial Agents and Chemotherapy. 2016;**60**(8):4610-4619

[69] Ismail A, Auclair F, McCarthy AE. Recrudescence of chronic *P. falciparum* malaria 13 years after exposure. Travel Medicine and Infectious Diseases. 2020;**October 2019**(33):101518

[70] Hviid L. Naturally acquired immunity to *P. falciparum* malaria in Africa. Acta Tropica. 2005;**95**:270-275

[71] Oboh MA, Oyebola KM, Idowu ET, Badiane AS, Otubanjo OA, Ndiaye D. Rising report of *P. vivax* in sub-Saharan Africa: Implications for malaria elimination agenda. Scientific African. 2020;**10**:e00596-e

[72] Fulakeza JRM, Banda RL, Lipenga TR, Terlouw DJ, Nkhoma SC, Hodel EM. Comparison of two genotyping methods for distinguishing recrudescence from reinfection in antimalarial drug efficacy trials. American Journal of Tropical Medicine and Hygiene. 2018;**99**(1):84-86

[73] Collins WE, Jeffery GM, Roberts JM. Aretrospective examination of reinfection of humans with *P. vivax*. American Journal of Tropical Medicine and Hygiene. 2004;**70**(6):642-644

[74] World Health Organization. World Malaria Report 2020: 20 Years of Global Progress and Challenges. Geneva: WHO; 2021

[75] Hwang J, Alemayehu BH, Hoos D, Melaku Z, Tekleyohannes SG, Teshi T, et al. In vivo efficacy of artemether-lumefantrine against uncomplicated *P. falciparum* malaria in Central Ethiopia. Malaria Journal. 2011;**10**:1-10

[76] Abreha T, Hwang J, Thriemer K, Tadesse Y, Girma S, Melaku Z, et al. Comparison of artemether-lumefantrine and chloroquine with and without primaquine for the treatment of *P. vivax* infection in Ethiopia: A randomized controlled trial. PLoS Medicine. 2017;**14**(5):e1002299-e

[77] Eshetu T, Abdo N, Bedru KH, Fekadu S, Wieser A, Pritsch M, et al. Open-label trial with artemether-lumefantrine against uncomplicated *P. falciparum* malaria three years after its broad introduction in Jimma zone, Ethiopia. Malaria Journal. 2012;**11**:1-11

[78] Yohannes A, Teklehaimanot A, Bergqvist Y, Ringwald P. Confirmed vivax resistance to chloroquine and effectiveness of artemether-lumefantrine for the treatment of vivax malaria in Ethiopia. American Journal Tropical Medicine and Hygiene. 2011;**84**:137-140

[79] Teklehaimanot A, Teklehaimanot H, Girmay A, Woyessa A. Case report: Primaquine failure for radical cure of *P. vivax* malaria in Gambella, Ethiopia. American Journal of Tropical Medicine and Hygiene. 2020;**103**(1):415-420

[80] Hossain MS, Commons RJ, Douglas NM, Thriemer K, Alemayehu BH, Amaratunga C, et al. The risk of *P. vivax* parasitemia after *P. falciparum* malaria: An individual patient data meta-analysis from the WorldWide antimalarial resistance network. PLoS Medicine. 2020;**17**(11):1-26

[81] Ariffin N, Islahudin F, Kumolosasi E, Makmor-Bakry M. Effects of MAO-A and CYP450 on primaquine metabolism in healthy volunteers. Parasitology Research. 2019;**118**:1011-1018

[82] Baird JK, Louisa M, Noviyanti R, Ekawati L, Elyazar I, Subekti D, et al. Association of impaired cytochrome P450 2D6 activity genotype and phenotype with therapeutic efficacy of Primaquine treatment for Latent *P. vivax* malaria. JAMA Network Open. 2018;**1**(4):1-12

[83] Zhou Y, Ingelman-Sundberg M, Lauschke V. Worldwide distribution of cytochrome P450 alleles: A meta-analysis of population-scale sequencing projects. Clinical Pharmacology and Therapy. 2017;**102**(4):688-700

[84] von Seidlein L, Auburn S, Espino F, Shanks D, Cheng Q, McCarthy J, et al. Review of key knowledge gaps in glucose-6-phosphate dehydrogenase deficiency detection with regard to the safe clinical deployment of 8-aminoquinoline treatment regimens: A workshop report. Malaria Journal. 2013;**12**(112):1-12

[85] Watson J, Taylor WRJ, Bancone G, Chu CS, Jittamala P, White NJ. Implications of current therapeutic restrictions for primaquine and tafenoquine in the radical cure of vivax malaria. PLoS Neglected Tropical Diseases. 2018;**12**(4):1-14

[86] Corder RM, de Lima ACP, Khoury DS, Docken SS, Davenport MP, Ferreira MU. Quantifying and preventing *P. vivax* recurrences in primaquine-untreated pregnant women: An observational and modeling study in Brazil. PLoS Neglected Tropical Diseases. 2020;**14**(7):1-16

[87] Daher A, JCaL S, Stevens A, Marchesini P, Fontes CJ, Ter Kuile FO, et al. Evaluation of *P. vivax* malaria recurrence in Brazil. Malaria Journal. 2019;**18**(18):1-10

[88] Siqueira AM, Alencar AC, Melo GC, Magalhaes BL, Machado K, Alencar Filho AC, et al. Fixed-dose Artesunate-Amodiaquine combination vs chloroquine for treatment of uncomplicated blood Stage *P. vivax* infection in the Brazilian Amazon: An open-label randomized controlled trial. Clinical Infectious Disease. 2017;**64**:166-174

[89] Commons RJ, Ja S, Thriemer K, Humphreys GS, Abreha T, Alemu SG, et al. The effect of chloroquine dose and primaquine on *P. vivax* recurrence: A WorldWide antimalarial resistance network systematic review and individual patient pooled meta-analysis. The Lancet Infectious Diseases. 2018;**18**(9):1025-1034

[90] von Seidlein L, Peerawaranun P, Mukaka M, Nosten F, Nguyen T, Hien T, et al. The probability of a sequential *P. vivax* infection following asymptomatic *P. falciparum* and *P. vivax* infections in Myanmar, Vietnam, Cambodia, and Laos. Malaria Journal. 2019;**18**(449):1-7

[91] Landre S, Bienvenu AL, Miailhes P, Abraham P, Simon M, Becker A, et al. Recrudescence of a high parasitaemia, severe *P. falciparum* malaria episode, treated by artesunate monotherapy.

International Journal of Infectious Diseases. 2021;**105**:345-348

[92] Wellems T, Sá J, Su X-Z, Connelly S, Ellis A. "Artemisinin resistance": Something new or old? Something of a misnomer? Trends in Parasitology. 2020;**36**:735-744

[93] Arinaitwe E. Artemether-lumefantrine versus dihydroartemisinin-piperaquine for falciparum malaria: A longitudinal, randomized trial in young Ugandan children. Clinical Infectious Disease. 2009;**49**:1629-1637

[94] Stepniewska K, Ashley E, Lee SJ, Anstey N, Barnes KI, Binh TQ, et al. In vivo parasitological measures of artemisinin susceptibility. Journal of Infectious Disease. 2010;**201**:570-579

[95] Degefa T, Zeynudin A, Zemene E, Emana D, Yewhalaw D. High prevalence of gametocyte carriage among individuals with asymptomatic malaria: Implications for sustaining malaria control and elimination efforts in Ethiopia. Human Parasitic Diseases. 2016;**8**:17-25

[96] The malERA refresh consultative panel on characterizing the reservoir and measuring transmission malERA. An updated research agenda for characterizing the reservoir and measuring transmission in malaria elimination and eradication. PLoS Medicine. 2017;**14**(11):e1002452

[97] The malERA refresh consultative panel on basic science and enabling technologies malERA. An updated research agenda for basic science and enabling technologies in malaria elimination and eradication. PLoS Medicine. 2017;**14**(11):e1002451

[98] World Health Organization. A Framework for Malaria Elimination. Geneva: WHO; 2017

[99] Rishikesh K, Saravu K. Primaquine treatment and relapse in *P. vivax* malaria. Pathogens and Global Health. 2016;**110**(1):1-8

[100] White MT, Walker P, Karl S, Hetzel MW, Freeman T, Waltmann A, et al. Mathematical modelling of the impact of expanding levels of malaria control interventions on *P. vivax*. Nature Communications. 2018;**9**(3300):1-10

Section 4

Viral Infectious Diseases

Chapter 6

Recombinant Interferon Gamma: Influence on the Cytotoxic Activity of NK Cells in Patients with Chronic Epstein-Barr Virus Infection

Irina A. Rakityanskaya, Tatiana S. Ryabova and Anastasija A. Kalashnikova

Abstract

NK cells play an important role in combating viral infections. In this study, we examined the effect of therapy with recombinant interferon gamma (Ingaron) on cytotoxic activity of NK cells. Sixty patients with chronic Epstein-Barr virus infection (CEBVI) were examined. All patients were treated with Ingaron at a dose of 500,000 IU every other day IM. Initially, they received 10 injections of Ingaron followed by a 10-day break to assess the dynamics of clinical and laboratory parameters. Then, the treatment was continued with five injections of Ingaron. In total, each patient received 15 injections or a total dose of 7,500,000 IU. The administration of recombinant interferon gamma at a total dose of 5,000,000 IU stimulated spontaneous and induced degranulation of NK cells in patients with CEBVI. After a full course of 7,500,000 IU of recombinant interferon gamma, CD107a expression on NK cells decreased but remained higher than before the onset of therapy and exceeded reference values. Thus, the maximum activity of NK cells in the peripheral blood of patients with CEBVI was reached 10 days after the administration of Ingaron at a total dose of 5,000,000 IU.

Keywords: NK cells, cytotoxic activity, chronic Epstein-Barr virus infection, recombinant interferon gamma, therapy

1. Introduction

1.1 Epstein-Barr virus

The Epstein-Barr virus (EBV) is a lymphotropic herpesvirus type 4 and the causative agent of infectious mononucleosis [1, 2]. The virus was first discovered and isolated in cells from African Burkitt's lymphoma by Epstein M.A., Barr Y.M., and

Achong B.G. in 1964 and later it was found that EBV is widespread throughout the world [3]. The first identified variants of EBV were type 1 (type A) and type 2 (type B). Type 1 (B95-8, GD1, and Akata) is the main type of EBV prevalent worldwide and type 2 (AG876 and P3HR-1) is more common in Sub-Saharan Africa [4]. EBV variants have different replicative properties and a person can become superinfected with two or more strains.

EBV infects most people during their lifetime and, after the acute phase, persists until the end of a person's life. The life cycle of EBV is characteristic of a virus with a large DNA envelope, consisting of phases of primary infection, latency, and lytic reactivation. The EBV genome encodes nine different glycoproteins (GPS) for envelope entry. Currently, 13 GPS have been identified, 12 of which are only expressed during the productive cycle of lytic replication. One of which (BARF1, a decoy viral colony-stimulating factor 1 receptor (vCSF1R)) can also be expressed during the latency period [5]. The tropism of newly released EBV virions is determined by the GPS envelope, which appears to differ depending on the host cell [6]. EBV infects B cells *via* the CD21 receptor, epithelial cells, and, less commonly, T or NK cells. Infection of B-lymphocytes leads to the preservation of the EBV genome as an episome.

The virus undergoes lytic replication in epithelial cells and establishes a lifelong latency in circulating memory B lymphocytes, periodically reactivating from latency [7]. Epithelial cells are the first to become infected, as EBV is transmitted to recipients *via* saliva. B cells become infected when EBV is released from the oropharyngeal epithelial cells [6, 8]. Lytic replication increases the pool of latently infected cells. EBV virions released from epithelial cells prefer B cells and EBV virions released from B cells prefer epithelial cells due to the composition of the GPS envelope [9]. EBV reactivation (lytic phase) under conditions of psychological stress leads to a weakening of cellular immunity and can stimulate EBV reactivation and replication by weakening the cellular immune system's control over viral latency. Chronic EBV reactivation is an important mechanism in the pathogenesis of many oncological and autoimmune diseases [10]. During the lytic phase, the full set of virus genes is expressed and a progeny virus is produced. Virions produced during lytic replication in epithelial cells replenish the viral reservoir in an infected individual and ensure the transmission of the virus in the population. During the latency period, the virus expresses only a limited number of genes necessary to maintain the viral genome (in the form of an episome in the nucleus) and evade the host's immune system [8].

1.2 Natural killer cells

Natural killer cells (NK cells) are a unique subpopulation of cells that lack antigen-specific receptors. NK cells have high cytotoxic activity and produce a large amount of interferon gamma (IFN-γ) when they interact with transformed or infected target cells [11]. The recognition process of target cells consists of the signals they receive from activating and inhibitory receptors encoded by the germline. As a result of these interactions, the identification or death of target cells occurs.

In the absence of inhibiting signal, continuous stimulation of activation receptors deactivates NK cells and reduces their activity. When target cells transform or become infected, the expression of HLA Class I on their surface may cease. Therefore, multiple NK cell receptors along with the presence of activated cytokines and cells that adapt and express various receptors in NK cell compartment promote responsiveness of these innate cytotoxic lymphocytes [12].

The activity of NK cells is also regulated by four additional mechanisms:

1. repertoire of NK cells;

2. activation by cytokines or priming of NK cells;

3. adaptive or memory-like differentiation of NK cells; and

4. licensing of NK cells.

There are 30,000 subpopulations of NK cells that differ in respect of inhibiting and activating receptor expression.

During Epstein-Barr virus (EBV) infection, NK cell expansion occurs in peripheral blood, and the cytotoxicity of NK cells to EBV-infected cells increases. The expansion of early differentiated NK cells lasts for at least 6 months [13]; however, the cells in this period stop to proliferate and acquire CD57 marker of aging [14]. A higher count of NK cells correlates with a lower EBV titer in peripheral blood, which suggests that the level of NK cell response depends on the clinical severity of the disease. It was recently demonstrated that induction of lytic replication in EBV-infected B cells leads to an increased destruction of NK cells. This may suggest that EBV-infected cells become a target for NK cells. It is assumed that NK cells have no significant control over the establishment of latency. Therefore, although the population of NK cells increases and is capable to kill target cells, no influence on the viral load during lytic or latent infection is observed. It was shown that NK cells play a crucial role in the control of herpes virus infections when the presence of viral antigens leads to the activation, proliferation, and accumulation of these cells in sites of infection [15]. Therefore, NK cells are an important factor in the control of initial EBV infection because they eliminate infected B cells and enhance antigen-specific response of T cells by the release of immunomodulatory cytokines.

1.3 Antiviral functions of IFN-γ

Currently, there are specific antiviral drugs, but there is no single approach to the treatment of chronic EBV infection. The antiherpetic drug must specifically inhibit the replication of the virus. The moment the virus evades the host's immune response, it is a potential target for chemotherapeutic effects. The higher the selectivity of the drug, the narrower the spectrum of its antiviral activity, since the drugs affect only the stages of virus replication. Drugs approved for the treatment of herpes simplex virus 1 (HSV-1) and 2 (HSV-2), varicella-zoster virus (VZV), and human cytomegalovirus (HCMV) are nucleoside (i.e., acyclovir (ACV), penciclovir (PCV), ganciclovir (GCV), and its oral prodrugs; valacyclovir (VACV), famciclovir (FAM), and valganciclovir (VGCV), respectively), nucleotide (i.e., cidofovir (CDV)), and pyrophosphate (i.e., foscavir (foscarnet sodium), PFA) [16, 17]. None of these drugs have received FDA (Food and Drug Administration) or EMA (European Medicines Agency) approval for the treatment of EBV infections [8, 18].

IFN-γ has a direct antiviral action on infected cells, and also activates local dendritic cells, macrophages, and NK cells, modulates differentiation and maturing of T cells and B cells, and promotes inflammation and antiviral functions [19]. Suppression of any stage of the life cycle of virus can suppress the replication of its genome during infection. IFN-γ is a powerful antiviral cytokine that disrupts the life cycle of virus in stimulated cells on various stages. There are several mechanisms of its action:

1. it inhibits virus infiltration on extracellular and intracellular stage by controlling expression and/or distribution of respective receptors;

2. it inhibits replication by disrupting the replication niche of the virus;

3. it disrupts gene expression by preventing translation;

4. it prevents the assembly of the nucleocapsid by affecting its stability;

5. it disrupts the release of virus by breaking the disulfide bridge, a significant part of cellular interactions;

6. it suppresses the main regulator of viral transcription and changes reactivation of viruses; and

7. it can inhibit the infiltration of invasive viruses on the stage of their transition from endosome to cytoplasm [19].

Some well-known antiviral functions of IFN-γ lack specific antiviral mechanism. For instance, IFN-γ strongly induces indoleamine-2,3-dioxygenase (IDO) and nitric oxide synthase (NOS). The depletion of tryptophan and the production of nitric oxide (NO) due to the expression of IDO and NOS have pronounced antiviral effects, but their molecular details generally remain unclear. IFN-γ can also manifest non-cytolytic activity against some viruses. However, specific targets and effector proteins of IFN-γ-dependent antiviral response are largely unknown [20]. Further studies are needed to clarify the antiviral mechanisms of IFN-γ, especially considering its strong immunomodulatory action.

In Russia, the only registered IFN-γ drug is Ingaron manufactured by OOO NPP FARMAKLON. It is obtained by the microbiological synthesis in recombinant *Escherichia coli* strain and purified by column chromatography. The molecule consists of 144 amino acid residues; the first three residues (Cys-Tyr-Cys) are replaced with Met.

The objective of the present research is to study the recombinant IFN-γ (Ingaron) action on dynamics of content of EBV DNA in the saliva sample, the killer cells content post-therapy, and changes of cytotoxic activity of the killer cells, and assess the influence of cytotoxic activity of the natural killers on the clinical complaint development and progression of illness in patients with CEBVI after the therapy completion.

2. Materials and methods

Patients. The study group included 60 patients with CEBVI (39 women and 21 men; mean age 34.64 ± 1.21 years). The duration of CEBVI was from first complaints to laboratory confirmation and the diagnosis was 2.85 ± 0.56 years. Forty-three patients (71.66%) had frequent exacerbations of antibiotic-resistant chronic tonsillitis in childhood, and 15 patients (25%) had a history of acute infectious mononucleosis. All patients had a differential diagnosis of CEBVI versus other viral infections (human immunodeficiency virus, viral hepatitis, cytomegalovirus infection), toxoplasmosis, helminth infestations, and autoimmune diseases associated with EBV infection. The diagnosis was confirmed on a previous stage by laboratory investigation and expert examination, and the patients were referred for the immunological treatment. Those patients, who received antiviral and immunomodulatory therapy within the last 6 months, were not included in the study.

CEBVI characterizes with a prolonged treatment and frequent recurrences with clinical and laboratory signs of viral activity (mononucleosis-like symptoms) that are described in detail in the literature [21]. Patients suffer from low-grade fever (37.1—37.3 °C), weakness, unmotivated tiredness, excessive sweat (especially at night), constant discomfort and/or pain in throat, lymphadenitis, swelling of the nasal mucosa with postnasal mucus drip, and stomatitis. Some patients have cough, skin eruptions, arthralgia, and muscle pain in body and limbs. Manifestation of conjunctivitis and otitis is possible. Neurological disorders such as headache, impaired memory and sleep, impaired concentration, irritability, tearfulness, and depressive tendencies may occur. Internal organs may increase in size (hepatomegaly and splenomegaly evidenced by ultrasound investigation) and a heavy feeling under the right ribs may be present. Some patients complain about frequent cold-related diseases and concurrent herpes virus infections. Many of these patients have a history of prolonged stress and psychoemotional and physical overload that exacerbates their condition.

This clinical study was performed in accordance with the World Medical Association Declaration of Helsinki: Ethical Principles for Medical Research Involving Human Subjects (2013); the protocol to the Convention of the Council of Europe on Human Rights and Biomedicine (1999); and Articles 20, 22, 23 of the Russian Federal Law no. 323-FZ on fundamental healthcare principles in the Russian Federation (November 21, 2011 as revised on May 26, 2021). The protocol was approved by the ethical committee of OOO Tsentr dializa Sankt-Peterburg, Fresenius Medical Care. All participants signed a voluntary informed consent. Patients included into the study had no other diagnosed infections, chronical diseases, or changed immune status that could affect the results.

Clinical methods included taking of history, data on previous treatment, and concurrent diseases. The clinical condition of patients was assessed traditionally with consideration of objective data and complaints at the time of examination registered using a three-point scale (0—no symptoms, 1—mild symptoms, 2—moderate symptoms, and 3—severe symptoms).

Treatment schedule. All patients received therapy with intramuscular recombinant IFN-γ (Ingaron) at a dose of 500,000 IU every other day. The course consisted of 15 injections. In the first phase, patients received 10 injections (5,000,000 IU) of Ingaron at a single dose of 500,000 IU followed by a 10-day break to assess the dynamics of clinical and laboratory parameters. In total, 500,000 units are the standard daily dose of the drug, which is recommended by the manufacturer. After that, the therapy was resumed and patients received five injections (2,500,000 IU) of Ingaron. Ten days after the last injection, the examination was repeated. In total, every patient received 15 injections (7,500,000 IU) of Ingaron (see **Figure 1**).

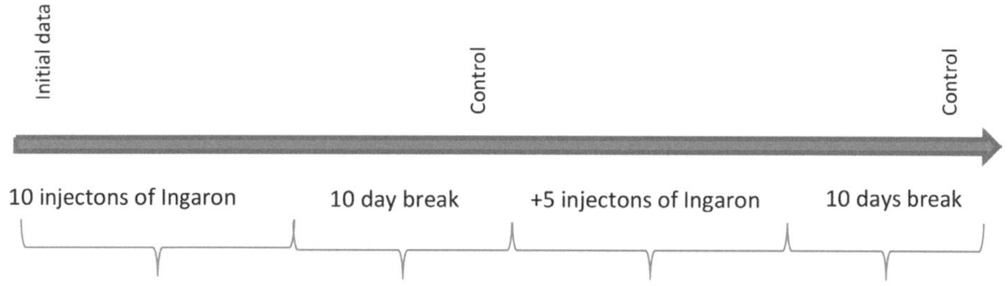

Figure 1.
Treatment regimen.

All patients tolerated the drug fairly well. After the first 3–5 injections, 14 patients (23.33%) had a fever (37.3–37.5°C), myalgia, chills, sore throat, and increased post-nasal drip. This was considered an exacerbation of CEBVI in association with the drug. After the seventh and eighth injections, these complaints fully disappeared.

3. Methods of examination using real-time polymerase chain reaction (PCR) with fluorescence hybridization

Viral DNA was detected in saliva samples using real-time polymerase chain reaction (PCR) with fluorescence hybridization, AmpliSens EBV/CMV/HHV6-screen-FL kits by the Central Research Institute of Epidemiology (Russia) were used. The unit of measurement used to estimate the viral load during DNA extraction from saliva is the number of copies of EBV DNA per ml of sample. According to the instructions, this indicator is calculated using the formula: Number of DNA copies = CDNA x 100, where CDNA is the number of copies of the viral DNA in the sample. The analytical sensitivity of the test system is 400 copies/ml.

Cytotoxic activity of killer cells was evaluated based on the spontaneous and induced expression of CD107a (LAMP, lysosomal-associated membrane protein on the cell membrane of lymphocytes, which is a sign of degranulation of lysosomes). CD107a was assessed after co-culture of peripheral blood mononuclear cell (PBMC) with target cells (K562, chronic human erythromyelosis). K562 cells express a range of ligands (MICA, MICB, ULBP2, and ULBP4) for NKG2D receptor of cytotoxic lymphocytes. The interaction between NKG2D and the ligands leads to the degranulation of lysosomes in NK cells, TNK cells, and lymphokine-activated CD8+ T cells, and to the expression of CD107a on their membranes. Therefore, the test reveals the ability of killer cells to participate in NKG2D-dependent cytolysis of target cells. Blood was collected in a vacutainer with heparin lithium as an anticoagulant. Sample preparation included separation of mononuclear cells suspension from peripheral blood using density gradient with subsequent washing, co-culture of PBMC and K562 in 10:1 ratio in a CO_2 incubator for 20 hours with anti-CD107a-AlexaFluor 647 monoclonal antibodies (BioLegend), and staining with anti-CD3-FITC/CD(CD16+56)-PE and anti-CD45PC5 monoclonal antibodies (Beckman Coulter). To assess the spontaneous cytotoxic activity, a respective volume of RPMI medium (Biolot) was added to PBMC suspension instead of K562. The samples were analyzed using a Navios flow cytometer (Beckman Coulter) up to 1,000 events in a minimum subpopulation of NK or TNK cells. The population of lymphocytes was defined as CD45+brightSSdim. The relative number of cells with CD107a expression (CD107a+) was assessed in subpopulations of NK, TNK, and T lymphocytes. The stimulation index was calculated as a ratio of induced expression to spontaneous expression of CD107a.

To assess the relative number of NK cells, multicolor flow cytometry was applied during the study of lymphocyte subpopulations in peripheral blood collected from the ulnar vena in vacutainers with EDTA. The samples were prepared according to the manufacturer's protocol. The following monoclonal antibodies were used: anti-HLADR-FITC, anti-CD4-PE, anti-CD3-ECD, anti-CD56-PC5.5, anti-CD25-PC7, anti-CD8-APC, anti-CD19-APC-AF700, and anti-CD45-APC-AF750. VersaLyse was chosen for the lysis of red blood cells. The samples were analyzed using Navios flow cytometer and respective reagents (Beckman Coulter) up to 5,000 events from the CD45+brightSSdim lymphocytic region. NK cells were defined as

CD3−CD56+ CD45+brightSSdim events. The absolute number of NK cells was calculated from the results of clinical blood analysis.

Statistical analysis. IBM SPSS Statistics ver. 26 software package (Armonk, NY: IBM Corp.) was used for statistical analysis of the data. Group results were presented as the mean (M) ± standard deviation (SD). Statistical comparison between groups of patients was performed using nonparametric Mann—Whitney U test. Differences in continuous variables were assessed using independent samples Student's t-test and were considered statistically significant if $p < 0.05$. Parametric (Pearson correlation) and nonparametric (Spearman's rank, Kendall's tau) methods were also applied. To check the independence of observations, linear regression analysis with the coefficient of determination (R^2), Durbin—Watson statistic, and analysis of variance (ANOVA) were applied. Fisher's exact test (F) was calculated to check the statistical significance of the model. A standard β coefficient with 95% confidence intervals was calculated. The threshold significance of differences in this study was 0.05.

4. Results

4.1 The effectiveness of treatment with recombinant IFN-γ (Ingaron)

In all patients (n=60), EBV infection was confirmed by PCR reaction in saliva samples. The study of DNA PCR was carried out 10 days after the administration of 10 injections of Ingaron (total 5,000,000 IU). After that, patients received five more injections of Ingaron (2,500,000 IU), and the number of copies of EBV DNA in saliva samples was assessed by PCR again. The results are shown in **Table 1**.

The data show a significant decrease in the number of EBV DNA copies in saliva samples 10 days after a course of 10 injections (5,000,000 IU) of Ingaron; 21.66% of patients had a negative result of PCR test. After a full course of 15 injections (7,500,000 IU) of Ingaron, 31.66% of patients had a negative result of PCR test of saliva samples (**Figure 2**). This means that the effectiveness of antiviral therapy confirmed by negative PCR was significantly higher after 15 injections than after 10 injections (p = 0.001).

4.2 Presence of NK cells in peripheral blood

The presence of NK cells in peripheral blood was assessed before treatment, after 10 injections, and after 15 injections of Ingaron. The results are shown in **Table 2** and **Figure 3**.

Group of patients	Copies/ml before treatment	Copies/ml 10 days after 10 injections	Copies/ml 10 days after 15 injections	P
	1	2	3	
Ingaron 500,000 IU, IM every other day	298331.57 ± 8326.80 (n = 60), 95% CI: 166707.75—435596.23	177369.51 ± 3994.40 (n = 47) 95% CI: 85699.01—326572.72 13 patients (21.66%) had 0.00 copies	8593.92 ± 3248.46 (n = 41) 95% CI: 2422.26—13232.15 19 patients (31.66%) had 0.00 copies	P1,2 = 0.0001 P1,3 = 0.0001 P2,3 = 0.001

Table 1.
The dynamics of the number of copies of EBV DNA after treatment with Ingaron in patients with CEBVI.

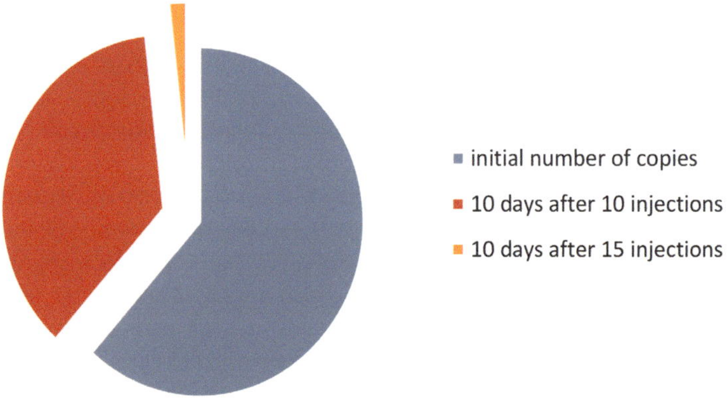

Figure 2.
The dynamics of EBV DNA in saliva samples before and after treatment with Ingaron in patients with CEBVI.

Subpopulations of mononuclear cells in blood, %	Before treatment with Ingaron	10 days after 10 injections	10 days after 15 injections	p
	1	2	3	
CD3−CD16+CD56+	10.95 ± 0.78 95% CI: 9.53—12.58	15.37 ± 0.96 95% CI: 13.59—17.28	12.33 ± 0.76 95% CI: 10.93—13.72	P1,2 = 0.001 P1,3 = 0.006 P2,3 = 0.001
CD3+CD16+CD56+	6.97 ± 0.63 95% CI: 5.81—8.16	9.46 ± 0.65 95% CI: 7.60—12.25	5.89 ± 0.68 95% CI: 4.52—7.18	P1,2 = 0.031 P1,3 = 0.328 P2,3 = 0.001
CD3+CD16+CD56−	2.97 ± 0,33 95% CI: 2.34—3.66	4.74 ± 0.56 95% CI: 3.64—6.20	3.89 ± 0.31 95% CI: 3.30—4.50	P1,2 = 0.001 P1,3 = 0.031 P2,3 = 0.04

Table 2.
The content of NK cells (%) in blood before and after the treatment with Ingaron in patients with CEBVI.

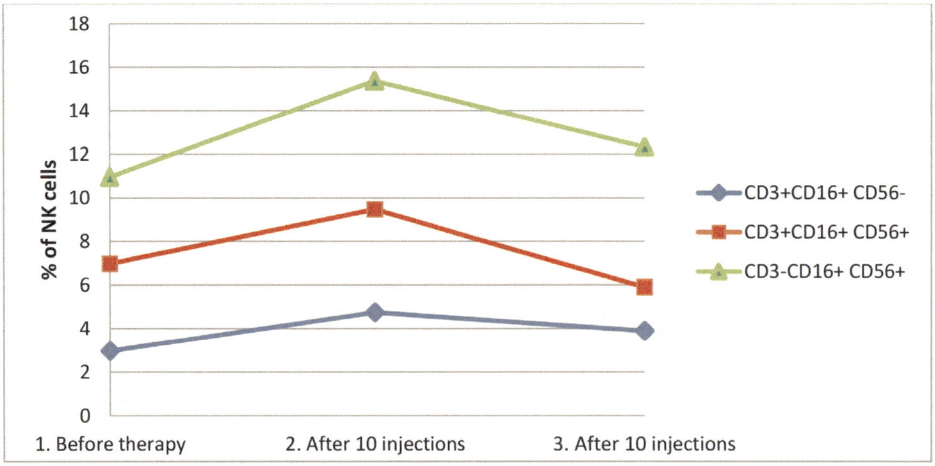

Figure 3.
Dynamics of the content of NK-cells (%) in the blood before and after treatment with Ingaron in patients with CHEBVI.

The data show that the presence of NK cells in peripheral blood is significantly higher after administration of 10 injections of the drug and decreases after 15 injections, but generally still exceeds the level before treatment.

4.3 Dynamics of cytotoxic activity of NK cells

Next, the dynamics of cytotoxic activity of NK cells before treatment and 10 days after 10 injections of Ingaron was assessed (**Table 2**). The expression of CD107a on NK cells 10 days after 10 injections of Ingaron significantly increased and exceeded referent values. This means that the introduction of recombinant IFN-γ at a total dose of 5,000,000 IU stimulates spontaneous and induced degranulation of NK cells and stimulation index in patients with CEBVI. After a full course of treatment (7,500,000 IU of recombinant IFN-γ), the expression of CD107a on NK cells reduced but was still higher than before treatment and exceeded referent values. Therefore, the maximum activity of NK cells in peripheral blood in patients with CEBVI was observed 10 days after administration of a total dose of 5,000,000 IU Ingaron (**Table 3**).

Expression of CD107a	Before treatment	10 days after the first stage of treatment (10 injections)	Reference values	p
Expression of degranulation marker CD107a on CD3−CD16+CD56+ cells				
Spontaneous	2.94 ± 0.35 95% CI: 2.31—3.72	5.22 ± 0.40 95% CI: 3.47—5.09	0.9—3.3	p = 0.001
Induced	19.20 ± 1.12 95% CI: 16.98—21.39	22.06 ± 1.09 95% CI: 19.22—3.50	11.0—24.0	p = 0.003
Stimulation index	11.05 ± 0.91 95% CI: 10.20—16.47	15.22 ± 1.05 95% CI: 12.17—16.45	5.5—17.0	p = 0.001
Expression of degranulation marker CD107a on CD3+CD16+CD56+ cells				
Spontaneous	1.46 ± 0.15 95% CI: 1.16—1.78	2.60 ± 0.25 95% CI: 1.52—2.50	0.4—1.6	p = 0.004
Induced	2.50 ± 0.26 95% CI: 2.02—3.02	5.01 ± 1.47 95% CI: 2.69—8.45	0.5—3.0	p = 0. 001
Stimulation index	2.27 ± 0.30 95% CI: 1.75—2.95	3.59 ± 0.58 95% CI: 2.54—4.80	1.0—2.5	p = 0.024
Expression of degranulation marker CD107a on CD3+CD16+CD56− cells				
Spontaneous	0.31 ± 0.02 95% CI: 0.25—0.37	0.71 ± 0.13 95% CI: 0.47—1.02	0.1—0.4	p = 0.009
Induced	0.34 ± 0.03 95% CI: 0.26—0.42	1.23 ± 0.18 95% CI: 0.88—1.59	0.1—0.4	p = 0.0001
Stimulation index	1.14 ± 0.06 95% CI: 1.02—1.28	1.62 ± 0.15 95% CI: 1.35—1.94	≤ 1.0	p = 0.002

Table 3.
The dynamics of the expression degranulation marker CD107a on NK cells, before treatment, and 10 days after 10 injections of Ingaron in patients with CEBVI.

Expression of CD107a	Before treatment	10 days after the second stage of treatment (15 injections)	Reference values	P
Expression of degranulation marker CD107a on CD3−CD16+CD56+ cells				
Spontaneous	2.94 ± 0.35 95% CI: 2.31—3.72	3.99 ± 0.41 95% CI: 3.26 — 4.86	0.9—3.3	p = 0.056
Induced	19.20 ± 1.12 95% CI: 16.98—21.39	21.08 ± 1.01 95% CI: 19.05—23.04	11.0—24.0	p = 0.02
Stimulation index	11.05 ± 0.91 95% CI: 10.20—16.47	13.08 ± 0.99 95% CI: 11.12—15.07	5.5—17.0	p = 0.0001
Expression of degranulation marker CD107a On CD3+CD16+CD56+ cells				
Spontaneous	1.46 ± 0.15 95% CI: 1.16—1.78	2.25 ± 0.26 95% CI: 1.74—2.78	0.4—1.6	p = 0.005
Induced	2.50 ± 0.26 95% CI: 2.02—3.02	3.39 ± 0.31 95% CI: 2.99—5.11	0.5—3.0	p = 0.04
Stimulation index	2.27 ± 0.30 95% CI: 1.75—2.95	3.62 ± 0.63 95% CI:2.82—4.00	1.0—2.5	p = 0.01
Expression of degranulation marker CD107a on CD3+CD16+CD56−				
Spontaneous	0.31 ± 0.02 95% CI: 0.25—0.37	0.51 ± 0.09 95% CI:0.34—0.72	0.1—0.4	p = 0.062
Induced	0.34 ± 0.03 95% CI: 0.26—0.42	1.08 ± 0.17 95% CI: 0.73—1.42	0.1—0.4	p = 0.0001
Stimulation index	1.14 ± 0.06 95% CI: 1.02—1.28	1.59 ± 0.13 95% CI: 1.35—1.88	≤ 1.0	p = 0.004

Table 4.
The dynamics of the expression degranulation marker CD107a on NK cells, before treatment and 10 days after 15 injections of Ingaron in patients with CEBVI.

Next, the dynamics of cytotoxic activity of NK cells 10 days after 15 injections of Ingaron was analyzed (**Table 4**).

The data from **Table 4** are shown in **Figure 4**.

The dynamics of the content of NK cells and cytotoxic activity visually resemble the sign "bell" or "arch" (∩) of varying severity. This direction of the obtained results indicates the development of a hyporeactive state of cells against the background of a longer administration of Ingaron (15 injections). The hyporeactive state of NK cells is a consequence of a decrease in the number of EBV DNA copies, which in turn is accompanied by a positive dynamics of clinical complaints after a full course of therapy (7.500.000 IU).

4.4 Dynamics of clinical complaints

The next stage of the work was an analysis of the frequency of the main clinical complaints in patients before treatment and after 10 and 15 injections of Ingaron. **Table 5** and **Figure 5** show the dynamics of clinical complaints during therapy.

Frequency of clinical complaints, %	Before treatment (n = 60)	10 days after 10 injections	10 days after 15 injections	p
	1	2	3	
Subfebrile temperature	83.33	45.00	36.66	P1,2 = 0.004 P1,3 = 0.001 P2,3 = 0.003
Lymphadenitis	50.00	46.66	41.66	P1,2 = 0.08 P1,3 = 0.052 P2,3 = 0.07
Sore throat	85.00	58.33	40.00	P1,2 = 0.001 P1,3 = 0.001 P2,3 = 0.001
Weakness	75.00	58.33	46.66	P1,2 = 0.01 P1,3 = 0.001 P2,3 = 0.05
Chills	71.66	68.33	50.00	P1,2 = 0.074 P1,3 = 0.001 P2,3 = 0.001
Excessive sweat	88.33	80.00	46.66	P1,2 = 0.052 P1,3=0.0001 P2,3 = 0.001
Swelling of the nasal mucosa with postnasal mucus drip	35	30.00	18.33	P1,2 = 0.08 P1,3 = 0.05 P2,3 = 0.07
Stomatitis	31.66	21.66	16.66	P1,2 = 0.05 P1,3 = 0.001 P2,3 = 0.07
Irritability and tearfulness	60.00	56.66	53.33	P1,2 = 0.058 P1,3 = 0.054 P2,3 = 0.072
Headaches, dizziness	35.00	31.66	30.00	P1,2 = 0.068 P1,3 = 0.052 P2,3 = 0.07
Impaired concentration and memory	40.00	38.33	33.33	P1,2 = 0.082 P1,3 = 0.056 P2,3 = 0.058
Disturbed sleep	41.66	38.33	35.00	P1,2 = 0.058 P1.3 = 0.070 P2,3 = 0.072

Table 5.
The frequency (%) of main clinical complaints before treatment and after 10 and 15 injections of recombinant IFN-γ in patients with CEBVI.

The data show that after the introduction of 10 injections of ingaron, there is a significant decrease in the frequency of subfebrile temperature, sore throat, weakness, and manifestations of stomatitis. After the introduction of 15 injections of ingaron, the dynamics of clinical complaints are more evident: a decrease in the frequency of subfebrile temperature, sore throat, weakness, chills, stomatitis, and swelling of the nasal mucosa with postnasal mucus drip.

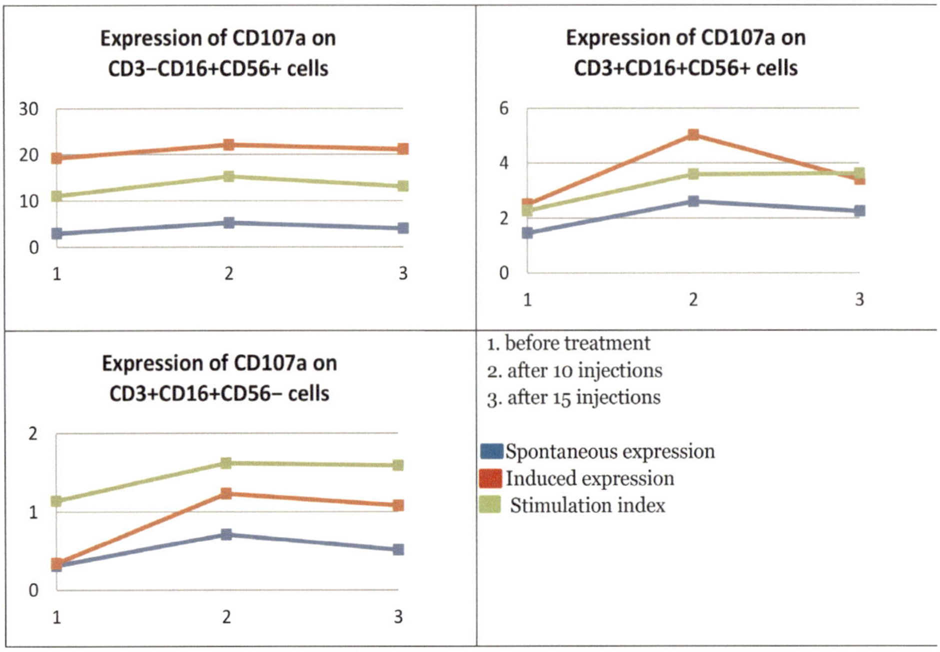

Figure 4.
The dynamics of the expression of CD107a marker of degranulation of cytotoxic granules by NK cells before and after 10 and 15 injections of Ingaron in patients with CEBVI.

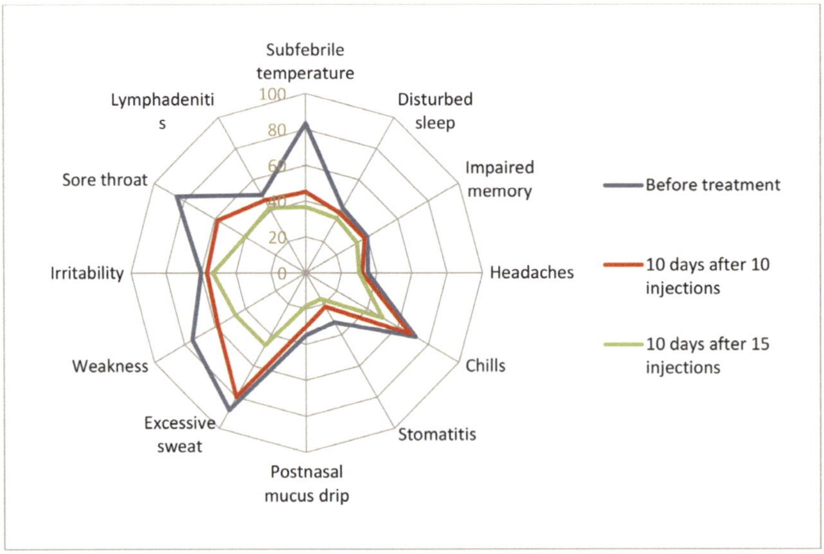

Figure 5.
The frequency (%) of main clinical complaints before treatment and after 10 and 15 injections of recombinant IFN-γ in patients with CEBVI.

4.5 Prognostic value of the presence of CD3−CD16+CD56+ cells in peripheral blood

To reveal the prognostic value of NK cells, linear regression analysis was performed with coefficients of determination (R^2) calculated using Durbin—Watson statistic, and also the analysis of variance (ANOVA), Fischer exact test (F), and standard beta coefficient (β) with 95% confidence interval. The results of the criterion F and the coefficient ß, indicating the significance of the obtained regression models, are presented below:

1. The content of CD3-CD16 + CD56 + cells in the blood before treatment contributes to the appearance of sore throat ($F = 4.186$; $p = 0.009$; $\beta = 0.457$; CI: 0.796; 4.237; $p = 0.022$).

2. The content of CD3-CD16 + CD56 + cells in the blood before treatment influences the development and progression of disturbed sleep ($F = 7.762$; $p = 0.007$; $\beta = 0.324$; CI: 0.773; 4.683; $p = 0.007$).

3. The content of CD3−CD16+CD56+ cells in the blood before treatment influences the development and progression of stomatitis ($F = 3.256$; $p = 0.045$; $\beta = 0.211$; CI: -0.187; 2.873; $p = 0.043$).

4. The content of CD3−CD16+CD56+ cells before treatment influences the development and progression of irritability and tearfulness ($F = 4.420$; $p = 0.039$; $\beta = 0.251$; CI: 0.091; 3.519; $p = 0.030$).

The results of linear regression show that the presence of CD3−CD16+CD56+ subpopulation of cells in blood before treatment is a predictor of the development and progression of clinical complaints in patients with CEBVI.

5. Resume

NK cells play a critical role in fighting EBV infection. NK cells are cytotoxic to EBV-transformed cells during the acute phase and limit the EBV viral load [22]. The mechanism of action of NK cells against EBV is not well understood. NK cell cytotoxicity is strongly activated by EBV-induced ligands on infected B cells. Activated NK cells use three main strategies to kill virus-infected cells:

a. production of cytokines;

b. secretion of cytolytic granules; and

c. death receptor-mediated cytolysis.

NK cells can prevent EBV entry into B cells and prevent B cell transformation via IFN-γ [23]. Human peripheral blood NK cells recognize EBV-replicating B cells by suppressing MHC class I surface molecules on infected cells [24].

The human NK cell compartment has up to 30,000 different subpopulations. Human herpesviruses promote the expansion of distinct subpopulations of NK cells, which then persist at an increased frequency for several months after infection.

During this time, they stop proliferating and acquire the aging marker CD57. Uncontrolled EBV infection develops with a decrease in NK cell compartments [25]. The hallmark of NK cell activation is degranulation, that is, the release of the contents of lytic granules. The granules consist of secretory lysosomes containing a dense core, various proteins, and take part in cytotoxic functions (e.g., perforin, granzymes) on the surface of the target cell. The inner surface of the granules is covered with CD107a (lysosome-associated membrane protein 1), a highly glycosylated protein that appears on the cell surface due to the fusion of lysosomes with the plasma membrane. Degranulation leads to the expression of CD107a on the cell surface and depletion of intracellular perforin. After degranulation, CD107a is exposed on the surface of the cytotoxic lymphocyte, protecting the membrane from perforin-mediated damage [26]. Resting NK cells, upon receiving signals for degranulation, are able to express surface CD107a and mediate cytotoxicity. Polarization and degranulation of cytolytic granules are two steps in NK cell cytotoxicity that are controlled by separate signals from different receptors. Neither polarization nor degranulation is sufficient for the efficient lysis of target cells. The ability of NK cells to kill virus-infected cells occurs before the "depletion" of NK cells, which is probably due to the depletion of cytolytic granules. The results of the NK cell degranulation analysis have been shown to correlate with standard cytotoxicity results. That is, CD107a expression may be a sensitive marker for determining cytotoxic activity [27].

In our study, the expression of CD107a degranulation marker on NK cells 10 days after the administration of 5,000,000 IU Ingaron significantly increased and excessed reference values. This means that the introduction of recombinant IFN-γ at a total dose of 5,000,000 IU stimulates spontaneous and induced degranulation of NK cells in patients with CEBVI. After the full course of treatment with 7,500,000 IU of recombinant IFN-γ, the expression of CD107a on NK cells decreased but was still higher than before the treatment and exceeded reference values. The maximum activity of NK cells in the peripheral blood of patients with CEBVI was achieved 10 days after the administration of a total dose of 5,000,000 IU Ingaron. Therefore, the results of the analysis of NK cells degranulation correlate with standard results on cytotoxicity as shown in studies by Alter G. et al. [27]. The expression of CD107a can therefore be a sensitive marker of cytotoxic activity of NK cells. The maximum expansion of NK cells in the peripheral blood of patients with CEBVI was observed after the administration of a total dose of 5,000,000 IU Ingaron, after additional five injections (2,500,000 IU) Ingaron, that is, after a full course of 7,500,000 IU Ingaron, the content of NK-cells decreased, but did not reach the initial level. The dynamics content and cytotoxic activity of NK cells visually resemble the sign "bell" or "arch" (∩) of a different curvature. In 1985, Talmadge, J. E. et al. were the first to demonstrate the bell-like curve of the dependency of NK cells presence on the dose of recombinant IFN-γ *in vitro* and *in vivo* [28]. They experimented on mice and showed that the activity of NK cells sharply increases 24 hours after the administration of recombinant IFN-γ and reaches a peak 48 hours after administration. The drug was several times more effective to increase cytotoxicity mediated by NK cells compared with IFN-α; its repeated administration led to a decrease in NK cells activity, and a hyporesponsive state developed. Preclinical and clinical studies of recombinant IFN-γ also showed a bell-like dependency on the dose when NK cells were induced by multiple or high doses of the drug [29]. This systemic hyporeactive state occurs not only in the spleen and peripheral blood, but also in NK cells isolated from the lungs and liver. In this case, the hyporesponsiveness of NK cells occurred when normal cells stimulated NK cells but the inhibiting signals from HLA Class I molecules were absent, or when excessive stimulation was stronger than inhibiting signals. Constant engagement of activating receptors and the lack of inhibiting receptors led to the hyporesponsiveness of NK cells.

Experiments on mice showed that the constant interaction of the activating Ly49H receptor with NK cells leads to the development of hyporeactivity of NK cells due to changes in the downstream signaling pathways from the receptor to the adapter molecule. The constant interaction of Ly49H receptor with its ligand *in vivo* results in a weak response of Ly49H+ NK cells to further stimulation from other receptors, whereas Ly49H−NK cells remain unaffected. Hyporesponsiveness of NK cells correlates with the suppression of the activity of Ly49H receptor on the cell membrane. When effective inhibiting signals are absent, NK cells experience sustained activation and become hyporeactive, which is known as the "disarming" model [30]. However, the most important mechanisms that lead to the hyporesponsiveness of NK cells need further investigation.

Based on the previously published results of studies on the mechanism of development of NK cell hyporeactivity and our data, it becomes obvious that long-term administration of recombinant interferon-γ in patients with chronic EBV infection leads to the development of a decrease in the function of NK cells. In our study, the development of a hyporeactive state of NK cells against the background of a longer administration of ingaron (15 injections) is accompanied by a decrease in the number of copies of EBV DNA in saliva samples and a more pronounced positive dynamics of clinical complaints in patients after a full course of therapy (7.500.000 IU).

The study of the inhibitory effect of pure recombinant human (rh) IFN-α and IFN-γ on EBV infection began in the late 80s and early 90s of the twentieth century. In 1986, Shigeo Kure et al. demonstrated that none of the rhIFNs lack pronounced inhibiting effect on EBNA expression in hidden EBV-infected Raji and Daudi cells. These results suggest that rhIFN act mostly on the early stage of EBV infection [31]. It was demonstrated in an experimental setting that pretreatment of Vero cells with either IFN-β or IFN-γ inhibits HSV-1 replication by less than 20-fold. Co-treatment with IFN-β and IFN-γ inhibits HSV-1 replication about 1,000 times [32, 33]. The authors proposed that a high level of inhibition after the introduction of exogenous IFN-γ was a result of a synergic interaction with endogenous IFN-α/IFN-β produced locally in response to HSV-1 infection. A study of the influence of purified recombinant interferons of all three classes on EBV-induced proliferation of B cells and immunoglobulin secretion showed that IFN-γ reduces B cell proliferation and immunoglobulin production if added 3–4 days after infection and that IFN-α and IFN-β effectively influence cell proliferation only within 24 hours. The authors showed that the antiviral effect of IFN-γ on EBV-infected cells is 7–10 times stronger than that of IFN-α and IFN-β [34, 35]. Our study demonstrated a significant decrease in the number of copies of EBV DNA in saliva samples 10 days after the administration of 5,000,000 IU of Ingaron, and the results of PCR test were negative in 21.66% of patients. After a full course of treatment with 7,500,000 IU Ingaron, 31.66% of patients had negative results of PCR test of saliva samples. This means that the full course of Ingaron is significantly more effective ($p = 0.001$). A strong and significant decrease in clinical complaints of patients was achieved after the full course of treatment.

6. Conclusions

1. Ingaron is a recombinant human INF-γ preparation. It has a pronounced antiviral effect, which is expressed in a significant decrease in the number of EBV DNA copies in patients with CEBVI.

2. After administration of a total injection of 5,000,000 IU of ingaron (10 injections), there was a significant increase in the content of NK cells, which indicates the effect of ingaron on the development of the maximum expansion of NK cells in patients with CEBVI. After administration of additional 2,500,000 IU of Ingaron (five injections), that is, when the course of 7,500,000 IU Ingaron was completed, the presence of NK cells decreased, but was still higher than before treatment.

3. Ingaron therapy stimulates spontaneous and induced degranulation of NK cells, that is, cytotoxic activity in patients with CEBVI. The maximum effect was obtained with the introduction of 5.000.000 IU of ingaron (10 injections) and it reduced after full course of 7,500,000 IU (15 injections) but did not return to initial values.

4. The content of CD3−CD16+CD56+ cells in the blood before treatment is a predictor of the development and progression of clinical complaints in patients with CEBVI.

5. The effectiveness of therapy in patients with CVEI, both in relation to clinical complaints and the number of copies of EBV DNA in saliva, is determined by the duration of administration of recombinant human INF-γ (Ingaron). At least 15 injections of 500,000 IU Ingaron every other day are required.

7. Future research directions

It is necessary to carry out further investigation of how Ingaron affects dynamics of content of other subpopulations of lymphocytes of peripheral blood in the course of treatment by the medication. Also seems to be interesting to study production of the anti-inflammatory cytokines (IL-1β, IL-6, and TNF-β) in the course of the Ingaron treatment.

Based on preliminary results of this study, we suppose that Ingaron possesses manifest anti-viral action and is one of the activators of immune response. The medication can be used as a combination therapy for chronic Epstein-Barr infection, which will save working population and reduce burden on the healthcare system.

Authors' contribution

Conception and research design—Rakityanskaya I. A.; material gathering and processing—Rakityanskaya I. A., Ryabova T. S.; data analysis and interpretation—Rakityanskaya I. A., Ryabova T. S.; lab research—Kalashnikova A.A.; statistical processing of data—Rakityanskaya I. A.; script composition—Rakityanskaya I. A., Ryabova T. S.; editing—Ryabova T. S.Kalashnikova A.A.; research supervision—Rakityanskaya I.A.; text writing and editing—Rakityanskaya I. A., Ryabova T. S., Kalashnikova A.A.; responsibility for integrity of all article's parts—Rakityanskaya I. A.; script further revision for important intellectual content—Rakityanskaya I. A., Ryabova T. S., Kalashnikova A.A. All the authors have made a substantial contribution to this study and approved the final script version.

Conflict of interests

The authors declare the absence of conflict of interests.

Data sharing policy

The statistical code, dataset used in support of the findings of this study are included within the article.

Financing

The study did not have sponsor's support.

Author details

Irina A. Rakityanskaya[1]*, Tatiana S. Ryabova[1,2] and Anastasija A. Kalashnikova[3]

1 Department of Allergology, Immunology and Clinical Transfusiology, Municipal Outpatient Hospital, Saint Petersburg, Russia

2 S.M. Kirov Military Medical Academy, Saint Petersburg, Russia

3 A.M. Nikiforov Russian Center of Emergency and Radiation Medicine, EMERCOM of Russia, Saint Petersburg, Russia

*Address all correspondence to: tat-akyla@inbox.ru

References

[1] Rostgaard K, Balfour HH Jr, Jarrett R, Erikstrup C, Pedersen O, Ullum H, et al. Primary Epstein-Barr virus infection with and without infectious mononucleosis. PLoS One. 2019;**12**: e0226436

[2] Dunmire SK, Verghese PS, Balfour HH. Primary Epstein-Barr virus infection. Journal of Clinical Virology. 2018;**102**:84

[3] Epstein MA, Achong BG, Barr YM. Virus particles in cultured lymphoblasts from Burkitt's lymphoma. Lancet. 1964; **7335**:702

[4] Kanda T, Yajima M, Ikuta K. Epstein-Barr virus strain variation and cancer. Cancer Science. 2019;**4**:1132

[5] Smith NA, Baresel PC, Jackson CL, Ogolla S, Toko EN, Heit S, et al. Differences in the Epstein-Barr Virus gp350 IgA antibody response are associated with increased risk for coinfection with a second strain of Epstein-Barr Virus. The Journal of Infectious Diseases. 2019;**6**:955

[6] Gunnar H, Nicole HT. Epstein-Barr virus and systemic autoimmune disease. Frontiers in Immunology. 2020;**11**: 587380

[7] Möhl BS, Chen J, Sathiyamoorthy K, Jardetzky TS, Longnecker R. Structural and mechanistic insights into the tropism of Epstein-Barr Virus. Molecules and Cells. 2016;**4**:286

[8] Graciela A, Erika T, Robert S. Novel therapeutics for Epstein–Barr Virus. Molecules. 2019;**24**(5):997

[9] Heldwein EE. gH/gL supercomplexes at early stages of herpesvirus entry. Current Opinion in Virology. 2016;**18**:1

[10] Kerr JR. Epstein-Barr virus (EBV) reactivation and therapeutic inhibitors. Journal of Clinical Pathology. 2019; **72**(10):651-658

[11] Spits H, Artis D, Colonna M, Diefenbach A, Di Santo JP, Eberl G, et al. Innate lymphoid cells–a proposal for uniform nomenclature. Review in Immunology. 2013;**13**(2):145-149

[12] Münz C, Chijioke O. Natural killer cells in herpesvirus infections. F1000Res. 2017;**6**:F1000

[13] Dunmire Samantha K, Grimm Jennifer M, Schmeling David O, Balfour Henry H, Hogquist Kristin A. The incubation period of primary Epstein—Barr virus infection: Viral dynamics and immunologic events. PLoS Pathogens. 2015;**11**(12):e1005286

[14] Tarik A, Anna L, Anita M, Seigo U, Vivien B, Karl-Johan M, et al. Role for early-differentiated natural killer cells in infectious mononucleosis. Blood. 2014; **124**(16):2533-2543

[15] Björkström NK. Strunz Benedikt, Ljunggren Hans-Gustaf. Natural killer cells in antiviral immunity. Nature Reviews. Immunology. 2022;**22**(2):112-123

[16] Poole CL, James SH. Antiviral therapies for herpesviruses: Current agents and new directions. Clinical Therapeutics. 2018;**40**:1282-1298

[17] Keith KA, Hartline CB, Bowlin TL, Prichard MN. A standardized approach to the evaluation of antivirals against DNA viruses: Polyomaviruses and lymphotropic herpesviruses. Antiviral Research. 2018;**2018**:159

[18] Xiaofan L, Akinyemi IA, You JK, Rezaei MA, Li C, McIntosh MT, et al.

A mechanism-based targeted screen to identify Epstein-Barr virus-directed antiviral agents. Journal of Virology. 2020;**94**:e01179

[19] Soowon K, Brown Hailey M, Seungmin H. Direct antiviral mechanisms of interferon-gamma. Immune Network. 2018;**18**(5):e33

[20] Jian Z, Ma R, Zhu L, Deng H, Li F, Zhao J, et al. Evasion of interferon-mediated immune response by arteriviruses. Frontiers in Immunology. 2022;**13**:963923

[21] Kimura H. Pathogenesis of chronic active Epstein—Barr virus infection: Is this an infectious disease, lymphoproliferative disorder, or immunodeficiency? Reviews in Medical Virology. 2006;**16**:251-261

[22] Chijioke O, Landtwing V, Münz C. NK cell influence on the outcome of primary Epstein-Barr virus infection. Frontiers in Immunology. 2016;7:323

[23] Jud A. Tonsillar CD56brightNKG2A+ NK cells restrict primary Epstein-Barr virus infection in B cells via IFN-γ. Oncotarget. 2017;**8**(4):6130-6141

[24] Zuo W, Zhao X. Natural killer cells play an important role in virus infection control: Antiviral mechanism, subset expansion and clinical application. Clinical Immunology. 2021; **227**:10872725

[25] Santosh K. Natural killer cell cytotoxicity and its regulation by inhibitory receptors. Immunology. 2018; **154**(3):383-393

[26] Dongfang L, Jose AM, Xufeng SW, Hammer JA 3rd, Long EO. Two modes of lytic granule fusion during degranulation by natural killer cells. Immunological Cell. 2011;**89**(6):728-738

[27] Esin A, Kucuksezer UC, Bilgic S, Erten G, Deniz G. Relationship between CD107a expression and cytotoxic activity. Cellular Immunology. 2009; **254**(2):149-154

[28] Talmadge JE, Herberman RB, Chirigos MA, Maluish AE, et al. Hyporesponsiveness to augmentation of murine natural killer cell activity in different anatomical compart ments by multiple injections of various immunomodulators including recombinant interferons and interleukin 2. Journal of Immunology. 1985;**135**: 2483-2491

[29] Talmadge JE, Tribble HR, Pennington RW, Phillips H, Wiltrout RH. Immunomodulatory and immunotherapeutic properties of recombinant gamma-interferon and recombinant tumor necrosis factor in mice. Cancer Research. 1987;**47**(10):2563-2570

[30] Key PN, Germino J, Yang L, Piersma SJ, Tripathy SK. Chronic Ly49H receptor engagement in vivo decreases NK cell response to stimulation through ITAM-dependent and independent pathways both in vitro and in vivo. Frontiers in Immunology. 2019;**10**:1692

[31] Kure S, Tada K, Wada J, Yoshie O. Inhibition of Epstein—Barr virus infection in vitro by recombinant human interferons alpha and gamma. Virus Research. 1986;**5**(4):377-390

[32] Sainz B, Halford WP. Alpha/Beta interferon and gamma interferon synergize to inhibit the replication of herpes simplex virus type 1. Journal of Virology. 2002;**76**(22):11541-11550

[33] Kevin D, Monica M-S, Cunningham Anthony L. Herpes Simplex Virus Type 1 interactions with the interferon system. International Journal of Molecular Science. 2020;**21**(14):5150

[34] Lotz M, Tsoukas CD, Fong S, Carson DA, Vaughan JH. Regulation of Epstein—Barr virus infection by recombinant interferons. Selected sensitivity to interferon-gamma. European Journal of Immunology. 1985; **15**(5):520-525

[35] Gujer C, Murer A, Müller A, Vanoaica D, Sutter K, Jacque E, et al. Plasmacytoid dendritic cells respond to Epstein-Barr virus infection with a distinct type I interferon subtype profile. Blood Advances. 2019;**3**(7):1129-1144

Chapter 7

Airborne Transmission and Control of Influenza and Other Respiratory Pathogens

Jacob Bueno de Mesquita

Abstract

Despite uncertainty about the specific transmission risk posed by airborne, spray-borne, and contact modes for influenza, SARS-CoV-2, and other respiratory viruses, there is evidence that airborne transmission via inhalation is important and often predominates. An early study of influenza transmission via airborne challenge quantified infectious doses as low as one influenza virion leading to illness characterized by cough and sore throat. Other studies that challenged via intranasal mucosal exposure observed high doses required for similarly symptomatic respiratory illnesses. Analysis of the Evaluating Modes of Influenza Transmission (EMIT) influenza human-challenge transmission trial—of 52 H3N2 inoculated viral donors and 75 sero-susceptible exposed individuals—quantifies airborne transmission and provides context and insight into methodology related to airborne transmission. Advances in aerosol sampling and epidemiologic studies examining the role of masking, and engineering-based air hygiene strategies provide a foundation for understanding risk and directions for new work.

Keywords: airborne infection, inhalation exposure, infectious aerosols, anisotropic

1. Introduction

Seasonal and pandemic influenza remain global threats. Seasonal flu kills up to 650,000 people each year and pandemics have the potential to cause millions of deaths and disrupt societies. Despite surpassing the 100-year anniversary of the 1918–1919 global influenza pandemic with a death toll estimated at over 50 million, present-day non-pharmaceutical prevention strategies—including engineering controls like germicidal ultraviolet technology (GUV), filtration, and ventilation—remain inadequately used to quell seasonal influenza epidemics and emerging pandemics as demonstrated with ongoing epidemiologic waves of COVID-19. Stringent social isolation remains an effective approach over the centuries but may only achieve population-level compliance for short periods of time. Testing, vaccination, and therapies are helpful but have not been available at the outset of emerging pandemics, and face issues of waning effectiveness as pathogens evolve, and logistical and social issues related to rapid production and equitable dissemination. It is widely appreciated that the quest for improved non-pharmaceutical controls and vaccines is dependent upon knowledge of influenza virus transmission via direct contact, large droplet spray, and aerosol inhalation and deposition along the respiratory tract. Increasing precision and confidence of quantified risks posed by airborne and other transmission modes support better design and evaluation of engineering controls and other strategies to reduce population spread. To rapidly identify airborne pathogens and continually update knowledge about airborne infection potential of evolving pathogens, there is a need for sentinel epidemiologic and bioaerosol sampling surveillance systems.

Influenza intervention trials showed that the use of hand hygiene and surgical masks to reduce contact and large droplet exposure resulted in only mild risk reduction among susceptible household contacts of influenza cases and may have facilitated more airborne transmission [1]. Human challenge studies have shown that infection initiated through aerosols, compared with nasal instillation [2, 3], required a lower dose and resulted in more severe disease. Inhalation of bioaerosols is likely important for other acute, viral, and respiratory infections and was convincingly implicated by airborne viral transport computational fluid dynamic models for a deadly SARS-coronavirus outbreak [4–6]. The capacity to directly measure the extent and intensity of transmission risk posed by bioaerosols represents uncertainty for which research is needed. Failure to quantify the contribution of exhaled bioaerosols impedes the advocacy for and effective use of control measures and facilitates population vulnerability during seasonal epidemics and pandemics.

William Wells described the quantum theory of airborne infection [7] whereby infection risk is described by exposure to infectious doses, or quanta (which is, more specifically, the dose that would infect 63% of those exposed), generated by infectious individuals over time. Studies quantifying influenza virus and SARS-CoV-2 virus shed into exhaled breath aerosols using a Gesundheit-II (G-II) bioaerosol sampler support an understanding of airborne contamination by infectious individuals, provides a way forward for precisely estimating airborne infection risk in terms of virions with infectious potential and genome copies measured by quantitative reverse-transcriptase polymerase chain reaction (qRT-PCR) [8–11]. Human challenge transmission trials offer one way forward to quantifying the airborne transmission risk between infectious and susceptible individuals with known levels of inhalation exposure to exhaled breath, paired with measurements of viral load in exhaled breath. Real-world study in congregate settings where exposure may be unavoidable, including in healthcare or other public gathering places offers another approach that may provide more generalizable findings, yet may be more logistically challenging to achieve valid estimates of exposure [12]. Yet emerging genomic sequencing methods that can identify viral mutations shared between epidemiologically linked individuals can confirm transmission chains and may offer clues to the specific mode of transmission [13].

Reliable prediction of airborne risk informs disease control efforts by providing information about the relationship between various levels of exposure control via engineering controls—air disinfection by GUV, ventilation, and filtration—and reduce airborne transmission. This information is needed to inform public health approaches and infrastructure design to provide appropriate air hygiene for mitigating emerging pandemic viruses before effective vaccines and therapies become available. This chapter provides an overview of airborne viral infection dynamics and control with a focus on the scientific underpinnings required for future epidemiologic study designs under which longitudinal surveillance of contact networks can revolutionize understanding of airborne infection transmission by pinpointing transmission routes and refining estimates of infection risk by airborne and other modes in indoor spaces. Results from this line of research provide key information for guiding the strategic use of prevention methods—especially air disinfection by GUV—to protect against seasonal epidemics and pandemics in shared air spaces and, in particular, among immunologically vulnerable populations.

2. Disease burden and public health impact

The Forum of International Respiratory Societies emphasizes that acute respiratory infections are the greatest contributors to the global disease burden, responsible for 4 million deaths annually. CDC reports that influenza resulted in 9–36 million illnesses and up to 56,000 deaths each year since 2010 in the US, with annual estimated direct and indirect costs of $87 billion [14]. Respiratory infections cost over $15 billion annually in the UK [15]. Globally, seasonal influenza kills up to 675,000 people each year and influenza pandemics have the potential to cause millions of deaths and severe societal disruption. The health and economic burdens are amplified in developing nations with less access to health services [16]. The devastating loss of life, the morbidity and economic losses from COVID-19, trends in spillover of pathogenic avian influenza to humans with pandemic potential, and an increasingly interconnected world, all create an urgent case for improved prevention methods.

Prevention of these substantial population health threats cannot rely solely on vaccines, which are often poorly matched to rapidly evolving strains. During pandemic, the lag time in the production and dissemination of vaccines leads to widespread vulnerability and underscores the need for interventions based on viral exposure reduction to interrupt transmission. It is widely appreciated that the quest for improved non-pharmaceutical prevention methods—including reducing exposures through building-level air disinfection—or social distancing, and vaccines are dependent on understanding transmission risk via contact, large droplet spray, and fine-particle aerosol respiration (i.e., airborne) [17]. Vaccine development benefits from an understanding of host-pathogen dynamics related to transmission mode. There is strong evidence supporting the critical role of airborne transmission, and it is well-recognized that infection initiated by the airborne route is likely to cause more severe symptoms compared to infections initiated by contact or large droplet spray [2, 3].

The US CDC typically has recommended protective behaviors such as washing hands, covering coughs, and donning masks to reduce contact and droplet exposure, but has provided little specific guidance related to air cleaning or respiratory protection (e.g., fit tested N95s) to mitigate aerosols that are capable of penetrating and circumventing surgical or cloth masks. Intervention trials showed that the use of hand hygiene and surgical masks to hinder contact and droplet exposure resulted in only mild risk reduction among susceptible household contacts of nearly 800 influenza cases and may have promoted a greater proportion of airborne transmission [1]. Furthermore, those most likely to be exposed to airborne influenza, due to the use of hand hygiene plus surgical mask, tended to present with more severe symptoms characterized by fever and cough. Despite some delays in intervention initiation and imperfect adherence, such trial conditions reflect realistic population usage, while randomization and robust sensitivity analyses support internal validity to the extent possible. Although implementation of masking and engineering controls such as

GUV, filtration, and ventilation are well supported by existing evidence, the state of the science benefits from investigation to better quantify airborne transmission risk and the extent of the effectiveness of GUV, filtration, and ventilation.

A clear, dose-response relationship between dormitory rebreathed air fraction and likelihood of retrospective, self-reported acute respiratory infection (ARI) was observed in a study of 3,712 students in Tianjin, China [18]. A separate airborne infection risk model suggested that increased clean air supply could effectively control population spread of ARIs including influenza but may not have much effect on highly contagious infections like measles [19]. However, this study used estimated values of influenza contagiousness based on an airplane outbreak [20], where there was uncertainty about outdoor air exchange, and all secondary influenza cases were assumed to be connected to the index. More recently a comparison of two university dormitories in Maryland, USA showed that compared with a dormitory with higher ventilation the dormitory with low ventilation had 4 times (95% confidence 0.69–163.02) the ARI rate, although the sample size of infections reported in the high ventilated dormitory reduced the ability to make more conclusive comparisons [21].

While modulating airflow and ventilation can influence airborne contamination quantities and human exposure, unequivocal evidence from exposure chambers demonstrates the inactivation of aerosolized respiratory pathogens including influenza [22], vaccinia virus [23], and TB [24] under exposure to upper-room 254 nm UV-C light (GUV), representing a highly effective strategy to interrupt airborne transmission. But whereas current control techniques are unlikely to be strategically deployed, improved characterization of risk by transmission mode enables the most effective use of existing control strategies and may provide health benefits knowledge to help catalyze investment by communities, government, and public health agencies.

3. The human-challenge transmission trial for quantifying infection modes

A meeting of globally recognized influenza transmission experts was convened by CDC in 2010 to address knowledge gaps about the relative importance of influenza transmission modes that are reflected in uncertainty about hospital care and general population prevention guidelines [25]. The meeting discussed possible animal and human transmission experiments and explored the possibilities of conducting epidemiological studies with engineering and/or personal protective interventions. Although there was great enthusiasm for studies of population infection surveillance with upper room GUV or other airborne control interventions, preliminary work in this area was lacking. Ultimately it was determined that a human challenge-transmission study with interventions to control for transmission mode, surveillance of aerosol shedding, environmental conditions, comparison of aerosol infectivity of experimental and naturally infected influenza cases would represent the most scientifically sound approach.

4. Aerobiologic pathway for influenza and other respiratory infections

An abundance of laboratory evidence substantiates the aerobiologic pathway for influenza and other ARIs and supports new epidemiologic studies of transmission. The aerobiologic pathway [26], consists of a) generation of particles containing infectious microbes from the respiratory tract or environmental sources, b) maintenance of infectivity and persistence in the air before reaching a susceptible host, and c) deposition in at least one vulnerable locus in the respiratory tract of the new host.

With respect to infectious particle generation, exhaled breath particles contain a respiratory fluid lining of the small airways and are generated by small airway closure and reopening [27–29]. A team led by Milton at the University of Maryland observed 218 half-hour exhaled breath samples from 142 symptomatic influenza cases and detected culturable influenza virus in 39% of fine-particle aerosols (≤5 μm) with geometric means of 37 infectious particles by fluorescent focus assay and 3.8×10^4 RNA copies by qRT-PCR (geometric standard deviations 4.4 and 13, respectively) [11]. Using a G-II bioaerosol collection device to sample natural breathing (including incidental coughs), this research clearly shows that influenza cases can generate many virus-laden particles. The same research team using a similar methodology detected SARS-CoV-2 in 36% of fine and 26% of coarse aerosols, while also detecting infectious viruses [10]. Others using the G-II showed that singing produced the highest proportion of positive fine aerosols, followed by talking and breathing [30].

Once generated, infectious aerosols maintain infectivity and persist in the air before reaching a susceptible host. The airborne movement of infectious particles has been implicated in human and animal transmission of influenza and other respiratory pathogens. Computational fluid dynamics and multi-zone models simulating a three-dimensional aerosol plume rising upwards and around an apartment building with a SARS-coronavirus index case predicted the location of secondary cases [4]. Noti and colleagues measured infectious influenza in aerosols that had traveled across a room [31]. Upward dispersion of aerosols with slow settling velocity has been confirmed by influenza. A transmission between infected guinea pigs housed >100cm below exposed animals [32]. Numerous ferret studies report similar results. The ability for airborne particles to travel and initiate disease was implied by two postal workers who became infected with Anthrax following a known release of spores and no other known exposures [33].

Biologically active airborne particles carry public health significance given the potential for prolonged suspension and scenarios of exposure before removal occurs or through recirculated air that has not been filtered or sterilized. Studies of biological decay in aerosolized virus maintained in a rotating drum demonstrated infectious potential for influenza [34] and coronavirus [35] after 23 hours and 6 days, respectively. Although the exact sizes of the laboratory-generated aerosols used were not reported, these studies demonstrate prolonged infectiousness in particles <10 μm. The rate of biological decay as a function of temperature and relative humidity has been characterized through laboratory manipulation of viral-laden droplets [36]; and through airborne simulations with bacteriophage Phi6, a surrogate for influenza and coronaviruses [37]. Reduced decay corresponded with lower droplet salt concentrations associated with high and low vapor pressures, consistent with epidemiologic observation of peak transmission during the hot and rainy season in the tropics, and the cold and dry season in temperate climates. However other research using aerosolized virus from human airway epithelial fluid suggests that the influenza virus remains infectious independent of relative humility [38]. This latter work may be more convincing given the use of a more realistic human model. The aerosol half-life of SARS-CoV-2 has been reported at 1.1 hours (95% CI 0.64–2.64) [39], with infectivity measured at 16 hours with potential for longer persistence under longer observation [40].

Inhalation of airborne virus and deposition at a vulnerable locus in the respiratory tract can initiate infection. A human challenge study demonstrated an infectious dose for inhaled influenza A aerosols as low as 0.6–3 $TCID_{50}$ [2]. A study of exhaled breath from confirmed influenza cases showed that 99 and 87% of particles were less than 5 and 1 μm, respectively [28]. This shows that exhaled breath aerosols are well within the size range to penetrate the lower lung. Fine particle aerosols exhaled from naturally infected influenza cases have been shown to carry infectious viruses [9, 11]. Given that, epidemiologic, laboratory, and challenge studies fail to definitively confirm human airborne transmission and produce valid risk models, there is a need for methods that maximize external validity to community settings and enable confirmation of transmission modes for a range of ARIs. Observation of community transmission provides an ideal platform to validate risk models that parameterize the aforementioned aerobiologic path—viral aerosol generation, persistence, and deposition—leading to valid estimation of infectious dose. Observation of exposed, asymptomatic individuals satisfies the concerns of Fraser and colleagues, which identified asymptomatic cases as key to pushing R_0 above one [41].

5. Studies of influenza transmission risk by mode and the anisotropic hypothesis

Hand hygiene and face masks have been assessed for their potential to reduce influenza transmission and gain information about transmission mode-related risk. Cluster-randomized trials with hand hygiene and facemask interventions found mild reductions in risk among intervention users (effect for hand hygiene and facemask groups, separately) that did not reach statistical significance [42]. This finding was consistent with those from studies performed in Hong Kong and Bangkok that showed the effect of hand hygiene plus facemask to be small at best [1, 43, 44]. A similar result was observed for crowded, urban households in upper Manhattan after 19 months of follow-up in 509 households [45]. However, a meta-analysis showed that hand hygiene plus facemask interventions were associated with a statistically significant 27% reduction in transmission risk [46]. Hand hygiene alone had no significant effect but showed a trend toward reducing risk under higher humidity and suggesting a predominance of aerosol transmission in temperate climates that is weakened in tropical climates. Given that facemasks have been assessed to reduce viral RNA copies contained in coarse aerosols by 25-fold and fine aerosols by 2.8-fold [9], if such reductions are associated with reduced transmission risk, then the meta-analysis findings make sense. Several other studies and review papers provide extensive evidence for the role of airborne particles in both influenza [5, 47, 48], and SARS-CoV-2 [49–55] transmission.

The hypothesis that influenza is anisotropic—that the route of transmission influences disease presentation [5]—is supported by early studies of human exposure to influenza contained in aerosols and nasal droplets [2, 3, 56], where aerosol exposure was more likely to result in influenza-like disease characterized by fever and cough, compared with nasal mucosa exposure representative of contact and droplet routes. The community-infected cases documented by Knight and colleagues exhibited similar symptomatology as Alford's infected volunteers, suggesting a natural tendency toward aerosol transmission. These findings were more recently borne out in ferrets where aerosol-infected animals not only presented with more severe symptoms but also shed more virus than their nasally-inoculated counterparts [57]. Similarly, cynomolgus macaques exposed to SARS-CoV-2 via aerosols were more likely to experience fever and severe respiratory pathology compared with those exposed via intratracheal/intranasal drops, suggesting similar anisotropy [58].

6. Findings from EMIT human challenge transmission trial

The human challenge-transmission trial (Evaluating Modes of Influenza Transmission [EMIT], ClinicalTrials.gov number NCT01710111) was designed to achieve an expected 40% SAR, however, achieved an actual SAR of 1.3% [59]. This finding on its own fails to provide definitive results regarding transmission modes, yet the low transmission rate from close-quarters exposure of infectious influenza cases over four consecutive 12–16-hour days with sero-susceptible individuals suggests that the contact and spray-borne transmission modes were not important contributors. Comparison of this result with the proof-of-concept study that achieved a SAR of 8.3% under much lower exposure time and ventilation motivates discussion about the role of ventilation and exposure to airborne pathogens [60].

Bueno de Mesquita and colleagues used CO_2 data from the transmission trial, and knowledge of aerosol viral shedding by experimentally infected primary cases (known as "viral Donors") and applied the rebreathed-air equation—a modification of the Wells-Riley equation—to estimate an infectious quanta generation rate and RNA copy number per infectious quantum [19]. This analysis showed that the particular group of exposed individuals where the single secondary infection was observed was among the group with the highest exposure to virus contained in the exhaled breath of the Donors to which they were exposed. This suggests that the transmission may have occurred through the airborne mode. Assuming this, the airborne quanta generation rate (q) (95% CI) for influenza in the controlled human transmission trial environment among infected Donors and airborne viral shedding Donors was estimated to be 0.029 (95% CI 0.0270, 0.03) and 0.11 (0.088, 0.12) per hour, respectively. The number of RNA copies per infectious quantum was 1.4E+5 (95% CI 9.9E+4, 1.8E+4). Given this quantum generation rate, and levels of viral shedding in a college campus community in dormitory rooms evaluated for exhaled breath exposure, the typical viral shedder presents a low risk of transmission to a susceptible roommate during three nights of exposure in a well-ventilated dormitory but a moderate risk in a poorly ventilated dormitory. Supershedders at the 90th percentile of fine aerosol shedding would present high risk even in the higher ventilated dorm. The effect of higher ventilation could be modeled using the rebreathed-air equation and typically points towards the need for levels of air exchange far beyond what might be achievable by ventilation alone, underscoring the importance of air disinfection by GUV and filtration to mitigate superspreading.

The next question is whether the EMIT human volunteers experimentally infected by intranasal droplets simulate naturally-acquired infections to a comparable degree. To address this question, the EMIT study included an investigation of community influenza cases presenting with influenza-like illness. There was a low probability artificial nasal inoculation would have resulted in the highest levels of symptom severity and viral shedding observed among naturally infected cases selected on the basis of febrile illness [61]. Findings from these analyses generate new knowledge about influenza infection, disease, and transmission and inform future studies aimed at improving our understanding of respiratory infection transmission dynamics and associated disease. There is limited data elsewhere about the extent of shedding as a function of symptom profile, although asymptomatic individuals have been shown to shed 1–2 $\log_{10}$ RNA copies fewer than symptomatic influenza cases [62]. The extent to which asymptomatic infections may be more representative of populations infected by upper respiratory mucosal exposure is unclear.

The computed infectious quantum generation rate enables the comparison between estimated exposure to influenza virus and infection risk. Thus, given levels of exhaled breath aerosol viral shedding and ventilation rates for indoor shared air spaces, the Wells-Riley equation can be applied to estimate infection risk. Of course, this assumes that the assumptions inherent in the computation of the q in the EMIT human challenge-transmission trial can be generalized to other transmission scenarios. The population of susceptible volunteers had low HAI and MN titres, representing above-average susceptibility to the general population, suggesting q may be overestimated. The computed q must also be interpreted with caution because it represents a point estimate, with confidence bounds generated by empirical bootstrap, given that it was derived from a single transmission event. The q for influenza in the challenge trial is relatively low compared with the few estimations done for other respiratory infections. Yet applying the EMIT-derived RNA copy to infectious quantum relationship to naturally infected influenza cases shedding the most virus among 142 mostly healthy young adults gave a q value of 630 [63]. Analysis of a super spreading event on an airplane suggested q or 100 for influenza virus, while q for rhinovirus has been estimated at 4 [19]. Careful epidemiologic investigation of an explosive measles outbreak in an elementary school showed q of over 5,000 [64]. Analysis of a SARS-CoV-2 outbreak in a poorly ventilated restaurant yielded an estimated q of about 80 [55], while a super spreading event at a choir practice led to an estimated q of over 900 [65].

7. EMIT trial limitations and questions for future work

The EMIT challenge-transmission trial, like Alford's challenge study with aerosol viral exposure, used a population with low pre-existing antibodies to the challenge virus subtype. Thus, these studies are useful for demonstrating transmission dynamics with susceptible secondary cases but lack generalizability to the general population with varying levels of immunity. That only one transmission event was observed in a Control Recipient represents a major limitation, as the mode of transmission cannot be well deduced, and the risk ratio represents the lower bound for infection risk and lends uncertainty to the confidence bounds. Nonetheless, the EMIT analyses attempted to a) learn what was possible about influenza transmission given that the study was unique in its design and the largest human-transmission trial conducted to date, and b) fully assess the limitations of the study design to inform future investigations. Numerous questions exist to drive future studies aiming to refine risk assessment and optimize population prevention strategies. Such questions include:

1. To what extent do climate, subtype, and engineering controls affect transmission risk while accounting for variability in human susceptibility to illness, and the concurrent deployment of administrative and behavioral interventions?

2. What is the optimal set of social contact networks and measured indoor air quality variables to predict observed transmission events in a contained community

setting (e.g., dormitories, military barracks, nursing homes, hospitals, schools, occupational settings)?

3. What epidemiologic strategies would best support the effective identification of exposure networks and confirm transmission events, potentially by infection mode?

4. To what extent does infection mode influence the immune response and subsequent viral shedding peak, temporal shedding patterns, and virion infectiousness, and to what extent does age, sex, prior infection, vaccination, and immune status modify these effects?

5. Could viral load quantities and community characterization sampled at different sites (lung-produced aerosols versus upper respiratory tract-produced mucosa) and times throughout the course of infection indicate the mode by which infection was initiated?

6. How do symptoms correlate with infectious viral shedding from the lung versus upper respiratory mucosa across age, sex, socio-behavioral factors, immune status, and subtype?

7. To what extent is aerosol shedding a function of viral concentration in the respiratory fluid of the distal airways and expiratory volume, and how might these relationships change with cough, speech, singing, and other drivers of expiratory particle generation?

8. Implications for study design

Findings from the experimental challenge-transmission model should be evaluated in studies of real-world epidemiology and population transmission dynamics. This way the potentially important contributions of other important variables can be assessed: a) immunity and shedding dynamics, b) socio-behavioral factors related to human-human interaction and exposure, c) overall well-being including psychological stress, sleep, physical activity, and diet [66], d) features of the built environment where exposure occurs including temperature, humidity, sanitary ventilation (combination of outdoor airflow, filtration, and GUV), and e) the role of other airborne exposures including particulate matter, ozone, and nitrogen oxides.

The advantage of the experimental trial in a controlled environment is that a relationship can be drawn between viral shedding quantity and subsequent secondary attack rates, giving a dose-response relationship. However recent advances in genomic sequencing and bioinformatics show a path forward for using molecular markers, in combination with epidemiological contact and exposure surveillance, to confirm transmission chains [67–69]. Sequences from identified transmission pairs may be able to give information about infection mode if viral communities evolve distinctly in the lung versus the upper respiratory mucosa. There is evidence that influenza may manifest as compartmentalized infections in the lung and nasopharynx [11, 70]. Airborne transmission likely involves viral communities produced in the lung, while contact transmission likely involves nasal communities, thus enabling a path to identify infection route that requires characterization. Considering the nasopharynx and lung as separate entities that carry the ability to infect independently, reconstruction of transmission chains in observed contact networks may be possible by analyzing shared variants [13]. Bayesian approaches can be used to infer transmission events for outbreaks that are not completely sampled and/or are ongoing [71].

A study that simultaneously monitored ventilation rates in two neighboring dormitories housing first and second-year students and respiratory infections among the population found a trend towards a higher infection rate in the dormitory with lower ventilation, suggestive of a relationship between inhalation exposure and infection risk [21]. This study also showed a gradient of exposure levels to exhaled breath between rooms in a corridor that could support epidemiologic investigation of transmission chains. Longer studies with larger populations should be done that combine contact investigation and sequence analysis to confirm transmission chains. Symptom assessment, specimen collection for quantification of mucosal and exhaled breath viral load, viral community, immune biomarkers, and other health-related factors related to stress would provide necessary data sources to assess the relationship between exposure and infection risk that could be modified by immunologic factors.

9. Conclusions and implications for public health practice

Although new studies are needed to refine estimates of transmission risk by various modes to understand the relationships between infection mode, dose, symptoms, age, sex, immunity, and environment, the existing state of knowledge is sufficient to support the scientific underpinnings of public health interventions aimed at reducing transmission and population epidemics through targeted airborne exposure control. At the very least, airborne infection preventive measures should be used as part of precautionary strategies to protect populations from loss of life and livelihood associated with emerging pandemics. In the case of influenza, it may be that the infectious generation rate of the average infectious aerosol shedder is low enough to pose an only mild risk under conditions with abundant sanitary ventilation but may pose moderate to severe risk under conditions of less sanitary ventilation (**Figure 1**). Fine particle aerosol supershedders may pose a substantial risk regardless of sanitary ventilation. Although they may be quite rare in the population, supershedders may account for most of the population spread as shown in the case of SARS-CoV-2 [72, 73]. Investigation of exactly how much of this risk can be attenuated by engineering controls opens the door for well-informed exploration of building design and operation strategies. That sanitary ventilation measures provide contribute to the control of any airborne transmitted pathogen represents a major advantage.

The magnitude of infection control measures required to prevent the community spread of airborne contagion is related to the infectivity of the pathogen (i.e., infectious dose shedding rate). Testing, quarantine, and isolation are critical measures to interrupt transmission by removing exposures to infectious sources and should always be considered. Yet there are challenges with achieving widespread access to sensitive tests for emerging pathogens, and compliance with quarantine and isolation procedures. Engineering controls including GUV, filtration, and ventilation provide an effective layer of protection that can be facilitated by the government as a social good requiring little if any behavior change or compliance at the population scale. Engineering controls—with an emphasis on GUV when dealing with highly infectious pathogens—can help move societies beyond reliance on social isolation and masking, especially given the social fatigue with these measures observed after more than two

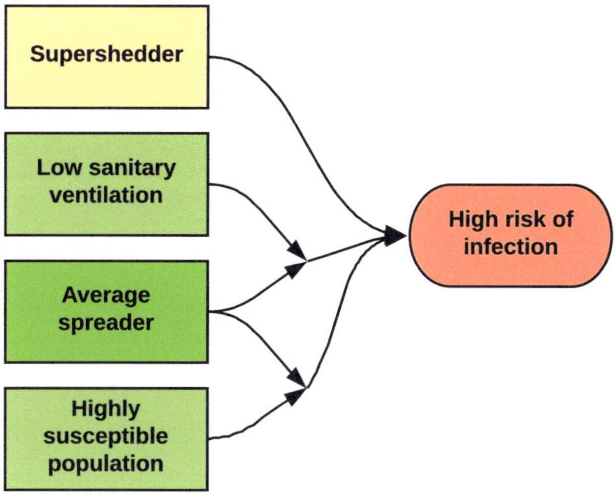

Figure 1.
Factors contributing to elevated risk of airborne infection transmission. Supershedders emitting high rates of infectious aerosol through exhaled breath or another aerosolization mechanism (e.g., aerosolization from toilet flush) can lead to high risk alone, or average spreaders can generate high risk under conditions of low sanitary ventilation or among populations of immunologically susceptible populations.

years of COVID-19 pandemic [74]. Vaccines and therapies are important measures, despite some problems with social acceptance. Yet, they take time to develop and deploy widely and may wane in effectiveness as pathogens evolve, and thus their use holds little bearing on the importance of engineering controls for population protection. Yet all available control measures can help as part of a layered approach and may be required for extremely infectious agents.

As demonstrated by Nardell and colleagues in the case of TB [75], and Bueno de Mesquita and colleagues in the case of influenza [63], there exist potential limits to the extent that ventilation controls alone can control transmission risk in shared air environments. Given that seasonal influenza epidemics cause substantial burden of morbidity and mortality, and COVID-19 and other emerging pandemic pathogens can exact an even more devastating toll, there is a great opportunity for wider use of infection control via engineering controls with the greatest effectiveness. SARS-CoV-2 subvariants appear to be increasing in infectivity and a super spreading event suggests that a highly infectious case could produce over 1,000 quanta per hour [65]. This compares with measles cases which may shed 500 to over 5,000 quanta per hour [19, 64] and an influenza supershedder who generated approximately 600 quanta per hour [63]. Yet upper-room GUV has been shown to mitigate measles spread in elementary schools [76–78] and provide many times the equivalent sanitary ventilation provided by outdoor airflow and filtration [23, 79, 80]. Newer far-UVC applications that allow safe exposure to the light directly have been shown to have similar levels or better air disinfection with potential for widespread use in a greater variety of settings [81, 82]. The use of GUV technology offers to reduce the theoretical limits of sanitary ventilation and lowers transmission risk in congregate settings where filtration, outdoor airflow, and masking may not offer sufficient protection.

Author details

Jacob Bueno de Mesquita
Lawrence Berkeley National Laboratory, Berkeley, CA, USA

*Address all correspondence to: jbuenodemesquita@gmail.com

References

[1] Cowling BJ et al. Aerosol transmission is an important mode of influenza A virus spread. Nature Communications. 2013;**4**:1-6

[2] Alford RH, Kasel JA, Gerone PJ, Knight V. Human influenza resulting from aerosol inhalation. Proceedings of the Society for Experimental Biology and Medicine. 1966;**122**(3):800-804. DOI: 10.3181/00379727-122-31255

[3] Henle W, Henle G, Stokes J, Maris EP. Experimental exposure of human subjects to viruses of influenza. Journal of Immunology. 1946;**52**(2):145-165

[4] Yu IT et al. Evidence of airborne transmission of the severe acute respiratory syndrome virus. The New England Journal of Medicine. 2004;**350**(17):1731-1739

[5] Tellier R, Li Y, Cowling BJ, Tang JW. Recognition of aerosol transmission of infectious agents: A commentary. BMC Infectious Disease. 2004;**19**(1): 1731-1739

[6] Tang JW, Tellier R, Li Y. Hypothesis: All respiratory viruses (including SARS-CoV-2) are aerosol-transmitted. Indoor Air. 2022;**32**(1):e12937

[7] Wells WF. Airborne Contagion and Air Hygiene: An Ecological Study of Droplet Infection. Cambridge, MA: Harvard University Press; 1955

[8] McDevitt JJ et al. Development and performance evaluation of an exhaled-breath bioaerosol collector for influenza virus. Aerosol Science and Technology. 2013;**47**(4):444-451. DOI: 10.1080/02786826.2012.762973

[9] Milton DK, Fabian MP, Cowling BJ, Grantham ML, McDevitt JJ. Influenza virus aerosols in human exhaled breath: Particle size, culturability, and effect of surgical masks. PLoS Pathogens. 2013;**9**(3):e1003205

[10] Adenaiye OO et al. Infectious SARS-CoV-2 in Exhaled Aerosols and Efficacy of Masks during Early Mild Infection. Clinical Infectious Diseases. 2021. DOI: 10.1101/2021.08.13.21261989

[11] Yan J et al. Infectious virus in exhaled breath of symptomatic seasonal influenza cases from a college community. Proceedings of the National Academy of Sciences of the United States of America. Jan. 2018;**115**(5):1081-1086. DOI: 10.1073/pnas.1716561115

[12] Bueno de Mesquita PJ, Delp WW, Chan WR, Bahnfleth WP, Singer BC. Control of airborne infectious disease in buildings: Evidence and research priorities. Indoor Air. 2021;**00**:1-32

[13] Worby CJ, Lipsitch M, Hanage WP. Shared genomic variants: Identification of transmission routes using pathogen deep-sequence data. American Journal of Epidemiology. 2017;**186**(10):1209-1216. DOI: 10.1093/aje/kwx182

[14] Molinari N-AM et al. The annual impact of seasonal influenza in the US: Measuring disease burden and costs. Vaccine. 2007;**25**(27):5086-5096. DOI: 10.1016/j.vaccine.2007.03.046

[15] Burki TK. The economic cost of respiratory disease in the UK. Lancet Respiratory Medicine. 2007;**5**(5):381

[16] Fischer WA, Gong M, Bhagwanjee S, Sevransky J. Global burden of Influenza: Contributions from Resource Limited

and Low-Income Settings. Global Heart. 2014;**9**(3):325-336. DOI: 10.1016/j.gheart.2014.08.004

[17] Erbelding EJ et al. A universal influenza vaccine: The strategic plan for the national institute of allergy and infectious diseases. The Journal of Infectious Diseases. 2018;**218**(3):347-354. DOI: 10.1093/infdis/jiy103

[18] Sun Y, Wang Z, Zhang Y, Sundell J. In China, students in crowded dormitories with a low ventilation rate have more common colds: Evidence for airborne transmission. PloS One. 2011;**6**(11):e27140

[19] Rudnick SN, Milton DK. Risk of indoor airborne infection transmission estimated from carbon dioxide concentration. Indoor Air. 2003;**13**(3):237-245. DOI: 10.1034/j.1600-0668.2003.00189.x

[20] Moser MR, Bender TR, Margolis HS, Noble GR, Kendal AP, Ritter DG. An outbreak of influenza aboard a commercial airliner. American Journal of Epidemiology. 1979;**110**(1):1-6

[21] Zhu S et al. Ventilation and laboratory confirmed acute respiratory infection (ARI) rates in college residence halls in College Park, Maryland. Environment International. 2020;**137**:105537. DOI: 10.1016/j.envint.2020.105537

[22] McDevitt JJ, Rudnick SN, Radonovich LJ. Aerosol susceptibility of influenza virus to UV-C light. Applied and Environmental Microbiology. 2012;**78**(6):1666-1669. DOI: 10.1128/AEM.06960-11

[23] McDevitt JJ, Milton DK, Rudnick SN, First MW. Inactivation of poxviruses by upper-room UVC light in a simulated hospital room environment. PloS One. 2008;**3**(9):e3186

[24] Riley RL, Nardell EA. Clearing the air. The theory and application of ultraviolet air disinfection. The American Review of Respiratory Disease. 1989;**139**(5):1286-1294

[25] Snider D, Bridges C, Weissman D. Meeting summary of the workshop 'Approaches to better understand human influenza transmission'. In: Presented at the Approaches to better understand human influenza transmission. Atlanta, Georgia: Centers for Disease Control and Prevention (United States of America), Tom Harkin Global Communications Center, Centers for Disease Control and Prevention; 2010

[26] Roy CJ, Milton DK. Airborne transmission of communicable infection--the elusive pathway. The New England Journal of Medicine. 2004;**350**(17):1710-1712. DOI: 10.1056/NEJMp048051

[27] Almstrand A-C et al. Effect of airway opening on production of exhaled particles. Journal of Applied Physiology. 2010;**108**(3):584-588. DOI: 10.1152/japplphysiol.00873.2009

[28] Fabian P et al. Influenza virus in human exhaled breath: An observational study. PLOS One. 2008;**3**(7):e2691

[29] Johnson GR, Morawska L. The mechanism of breath aerosol formation. Journal of Aerosol Medicine and Pulmonary Drug Delivery. 2009;**22**(3):229-237. DOI: 10.1089/jamp.2008.0720

[30] Coleman KK et al. Viral load of SARS-CoV-2 in respiratory aerosols emitted by COVID-19 patients while breathing, talking, and singing. Cold Spring Harbor. 2021;**74**:1722-1728. DOI: 10.1101/2021.07.15.21260561

[31] Noti JD et al. Detection of infectious influenza virus in cough aerosols generated in a simulated patient examination room. Clinical Infectious Diseases. 2012;**54**(11):1569-1577. DOI: 10.1093/cid/cis237

[32] Mubareka S, Lowen AC, Steel J, Coates AL, García-Sastre A, Palese P. Transmission of influenza virus via aerosols and fomites in the guinea pig model. The Journal of Infectious Diseases. 2009;**199**(6):858-865

[33] Fennelly KP, Davidow AL, Miller SL, Connell N, Ellner JJ. Airborne infection with Bacillus anthracis--from mills to mail. Emerging Infectious Diseases. 2004;**10**:996-1002

[34] Harper GJ. Airborne micro-organisms: Survival tests with four viruses. Journal of Hygiene. 1961;**59**(4):479-486

[35] Ijaz MK, Brunner AH, Sattar SA, Nair RC, Johnson-Lussenburg CM. Survival characteristics of airborne human coronavirus 229E. The Journal of General Virology. 1985;**66**(Pt 12): 2743-2748

[36] Yang W, Elankumaran S, Marr LC. Relationship between humidity and influenza A viability in droplets and implications for influenza's seasonality. PLOS ONE. 2012;7(10):e46789

[37] Prussin AJ, Schwake DO, Lin K, Gallagher DL, Buttling L, Marr LC. Survival of the enveloped virus Phi6 in droplets as a function of relative humidity, absolute humidity, and temperature. Applied Environmental Microbiology. 2018;**7**(10):e46789

[38] Kormuth KA et al. Influenza virus infectivity is retained in aerosols and droplets independent of relative humidity. The Journal of Infectious Diseases. 2018;**218**(5):739-747. DOI: 10.1093/infdis/jiy221

[39] van Doremalen N et al. Aerosol and Surface Stability of SARS-CoV-2 as Compared with SARS-CoV-1. New England Journal of Medicine. 2020;**328**(16):16

[40] Fears AC et al. Persistence of severe acute respiratory syndrome coronavirus 2 in aerosol suspensions. Emerging Infectious Disease. 2020;**2**(9)

[41] Fraser C, Riley S, Anderson RM, Ferguson NM. Factors that make an infectious disease outbreak controllable. Proceedings of the National Academy of Sciences of the United States of America. 2004;**101**(16):6146-6151. DOI: 10.1073/pnas.0307506101

[42] Aiello AE, Perez V, Coulborn RM, Davis BM, Uddin M, Monto AS. Facemasks, hand hygiene, and influenza among young adults: A randomized intervention trial. PLoS ONE. 2012;**7**(1):1-8. DOI: 10.1371/journal.pone.0029744

[43] Cowling BJ et al. Facemasks and hand hygiene to prevent influenza transmission in households: A cluster randomized trial. Annals of Internal Medicine. 2009;**151**(7):437-446. DOI: 10.7326/0003-4819-151-7-200910060-00142

[44] Simmerman JM et al. Findings from a household randomized controlled trial of hand washing and face masks to reduce influenza transmission in Bangkok, Thailand. Influenza and Other Respiratory Viruses. 2011;**5**(4):256-267. DOI: 10.1111/j.1750-2659.2011.00205.x

[45] Larson EL, Ferng Y, Wong-McLoughlin J, Wang S, Haber M, Morse SS. Impact of non-pharmaceutical interventions on URIs and influenza in crowded, urban households. Public Health Reports. 2010;**2010**:178-191

[46] Wong VWY, Cowling BJ, Aiello AE. Hand hygiene and risk of influenza virus infections in the community: A systematic review and meta-analysis. Epidemiology and Infection. 2014;**142**(5):922-932. DOI: 10.1017/S095026881400003X

[47] Nikitin N, Petrova E, Trifonova E, Karpova O. Influenza virus aerosols in the air and their infectiousness. Adv. Virol. 2014;**2014**:859090. DOI: 10.1155/2014/859090

[48] Tellier R. Aerosol transmission of influenza A virus: A review of new studies. Journal of Royal Society Interface. 2009;**6**(Suppl. 6):S783-S790. DOI: 10.1098/rsif.2009.0302.focus

[49] Morawska L, Milton DK. It is time to address airborne transmission of coronavirus disease 2019 (COVID-19). Clinical Infectious Diseases. 2020;**71**(9): 2311-2313. DOI: 10.1093/cid/ciaa939

[50] Greenhalgh T, Jimenez JL, Prather KA, Tufekci Z, Fisman D, Schooley R. Ten scientific reasons in support of airborne transmission of SARS-CoV-2. The Lancet. 2021;**397**: 1603-1605. DOI: 10.1016/S0140-6736(21)00869-2

[51] Kwon KS, Park JI, Park YJ, Jung DM, Ryu KW, Lee JH. Evidence of long-distance droplet transmission of SARS-CoV-2 by direct air flow in a restaurant in Korea. Journal of Korean Medical Science. 2020;**35**(46):e415

[52] Katelaris AL et al. Epidemiologic evidence for airborne transmission of SARS-CoV-2 during Church Singing, Australia, 2020. Emerging Infectious Diseases. 2021;**27**(6):e415

[53] Hamner L. High SARS-CoV-2 Attack Rate Following Exposure at a Choir Practice — Skagit County, Washington, March 2020. MMWR Morbidity, Mortality and Weekly Report. 2020;**69**:1-5

[54] Shen Y et al. Community outbreak investigation of SARS-CoV-2 transmission among bus riders in Eastern China. JAMA Internal Medicine. 2020;**180**:1665-1671. DOI: 10.1001/jamainternmed.2020.5225

[55] Li Y et al. Probable airborne transmission of SARS-CoV-2 in a poorly ventilated restaurant. Building and Environment. 2021;**196**:107788. DOI: 10.1016/j.buildenv.2021.107788

[56] Knight V et al. New Research on Influenza: Studies with Normal Volunteers: Combined Clinical Staff Conference at the National Institutes of Health. Annals of Internal Medicine. 1965;**62**:1307-1325. DOI: 10.7326/0003-4819-62-6-1307

[57] Gustin KM et al. Influenza virus aerosol exposure and analytical system for ferrets. Proceedings of the National Academy of Sciences of the United States of America. 2011;**108**(20):8432-8437. DOI: 10.1073/pnas.1100768108

[58] Bixler SL et al. Exposure route influences disease severity in the COVID-19 cynomolgus macaque model. Viruses. 2022;**14**(5). DOI: 10.3390/v14051013

[59] Nguyen-Van-Tam JS et al. Minimal transmission in an influenza A (H3N2) human challenge-transmission model within a controlled exposure environment. PLoS Pathogens. 2020;**16**(7):e1008704

[60] Killingley B et al. Use of a human influenza challenge model to assess person-to-person transmission: Proof-of-concept study. The Journal of Infectious Diseases. 2012;**205**(1):35-43

[61] Bueno de Mesquita PJ et al. Influenza A (H3) illness and viral aerosol shedding

from symptomatic naturally infected and experimentally infected cases. Influenza and Other Respiratory Viruses. 2021;**15**(1):154-163. DOI: 10.1111/irv.12790

[62] Ip DKM et al. Viral shedding and transmission potential of asymptomatic and paucisymptomatic influenza virus infections in the community. Clinical Infectious Diseases. 2017;**64**(6):736-742

[63] Bueno de Mesquita PJ, Noakes CJ, Milton DK. Quantitative aerobiologic analysis of an influenza human challenge-transmission trial. Indoor Air. 2020;**30**(6):1189-1198. DOI: 10.1111/ina.12701

[64] Riley EC, Murphy G, Riley RL. Airborne spread of measles in a suburban elementary school. American Journal of Epidemiology. 1978;**107**(5):421-432. DOI: 10.1093/oxfordjournals.aje.a112560

[65] Miller SL et al. Transmission of SARS-CoV-2 by inhalation of respiratory aerosol in the Skagit Valley Chorale superspreading event. Indoor Air. 2020;**31**:314-323. DOI: 10.1111/ina.12751

[66] Cohen S, Tyrrell DA, Smith AP. Psychological stress and susceptibility to the common cold. The New England Journal of Medicine. 1991;**325**(9):606-612. DOI: 10.1056/NEJM199108293250903

[67] Campbell F, Cori A, Ferguson N, Jombart T. Bayesian inference of transmission chains using timing of symptoms, pathogen genomes and contact data. PLoS Computational Biology. 2019;**15**(3):e1006930

[68] Volz EM, Pond SLK, Ward MJ, Brown AJL, Frost SDW. Phylodynamics of infectious disease epidemics. Genetics. 2009;**183**(4):1421-1430. DOI: 10.1534/genetics.109.106021

[69] Volz EM, Frost SDW. Inferring the source of transmission with phylogenetic data. PLoS Computing. 2013;**9**(12):e1003397

[70] Piralla A et al. Segregation of virulent influenza A(H1N1) variants in the lower respiratory tract of critically ill patients during the 2010-2011 seasonal epidemic. PloS One. 2011;**6**(12):e28332

[71] Didelot X, Fraser C, Gardy J, Colijn C. Genomic infectious disease epidemiology in partially sampled and ongoing outbreaks. Molecular Biology Evolution. 2017;**34**(4):997

[72] Adam DC et al. Clustering and superspreading potential of SARS-CoV-2 infections in Hong Kong. Nature Medicine. 2020;**26**(11):1714-1719. DOI: 10.1038/s41591-020-1092-0

[73] Endo A, Centre for the Mathematical Modelling of Infectious Diseases COVID-19 Working Group. Estimating the overdispersion in COVID-19 transmission using outbreak sizes outside China. Wellcome Open Research. 2020;**5**:67

[74] Sehgal NJ, Milton DK. Applying the hierarchy of controls: What occupational safety can teach us about safely navigating the next phase of the global COVID-19 pandemic. Frontiers in Public Health. 2021;**9**:747894. DOI: 10.3389/fpubh.2021.747894

[75] Nardell EA, Keegan J, Cheney SA, Etkind SC. Airborne infection. Theoretical limits of protection achievable by building ventilation. The American Review of Respiratory Disease. 1991;**144**(2):302-306. DOI: 10.1164/ajrccm/144.2.302

[76] Wells WF, Wells MW, Wilder TS. The environmental control of epidemic contagion I. An epidemiologic study

of radiant disinfection of air in day schools. American Journal of Hygiene. 1942;**35**:97-121

[77] Wells MW, Holla WA. Ventilation in the flow of measles and chickenpox through a community. Journal of the American Medical Association. 1950;**142**(17):1337-1344. DOI: 10.1001/jama.1950.02910350007004

[78] Riley RL, O'Grady F. Airborne Infection, Transmission and Control. New York: Macmillan; 1961

[79] Mphaphlele M et al. Controlled trial of upper room ultraviolet air disinfection: A basis for new dosing guidelines. American Journal of Respiratory and Critical Care Medicine. 2015;**192**(4):477-484. DOI: 10.1164/rccm.201501-0060OC

[80] Nardell EA. Air disinfection for airborne infection control with a focus on COVID-19: Why Germicidal UV is Essential. Photochemistry and Photobiology. 2021;**97**(3):493-497. DOI: 10.1111/php.13421

[81] Eadie E et al. Far-UVC (222 nm) efficiently inactivates an airborne pathogen in a room-sized chamber. Scientific Reports. 2022;**12**(1):4373

[82] Buonanno M, Welch P, Shuryak I, Brenner DJ. Far-UVC light efficiently and safely inactivates airborne human coronaviruses. Scientific Reports. 2020;**10**(1):10285. DOI: 10.1038/s41598-020-67211-2